I0824189

Eating Well *in Your Prime*

Hélène Mailleux
NATUROPATH

Eating Well in *Your Prime*

70 Natural Recipes
for Women's Hormone Health, Midlife, and Menopause

PHOTOGRAPHY BY
Atelier Chez Elles

ILLUSTRATIONS BY
Léa Morineau

TRANSLATED BY
Grace McQuillan

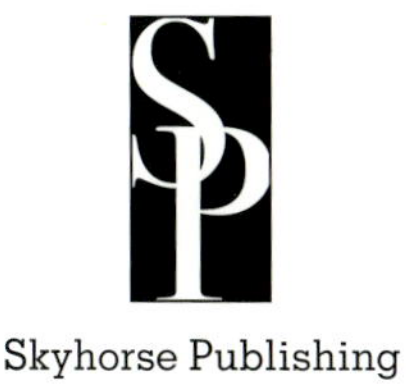

Skyhorse Publishing

CONTENTS

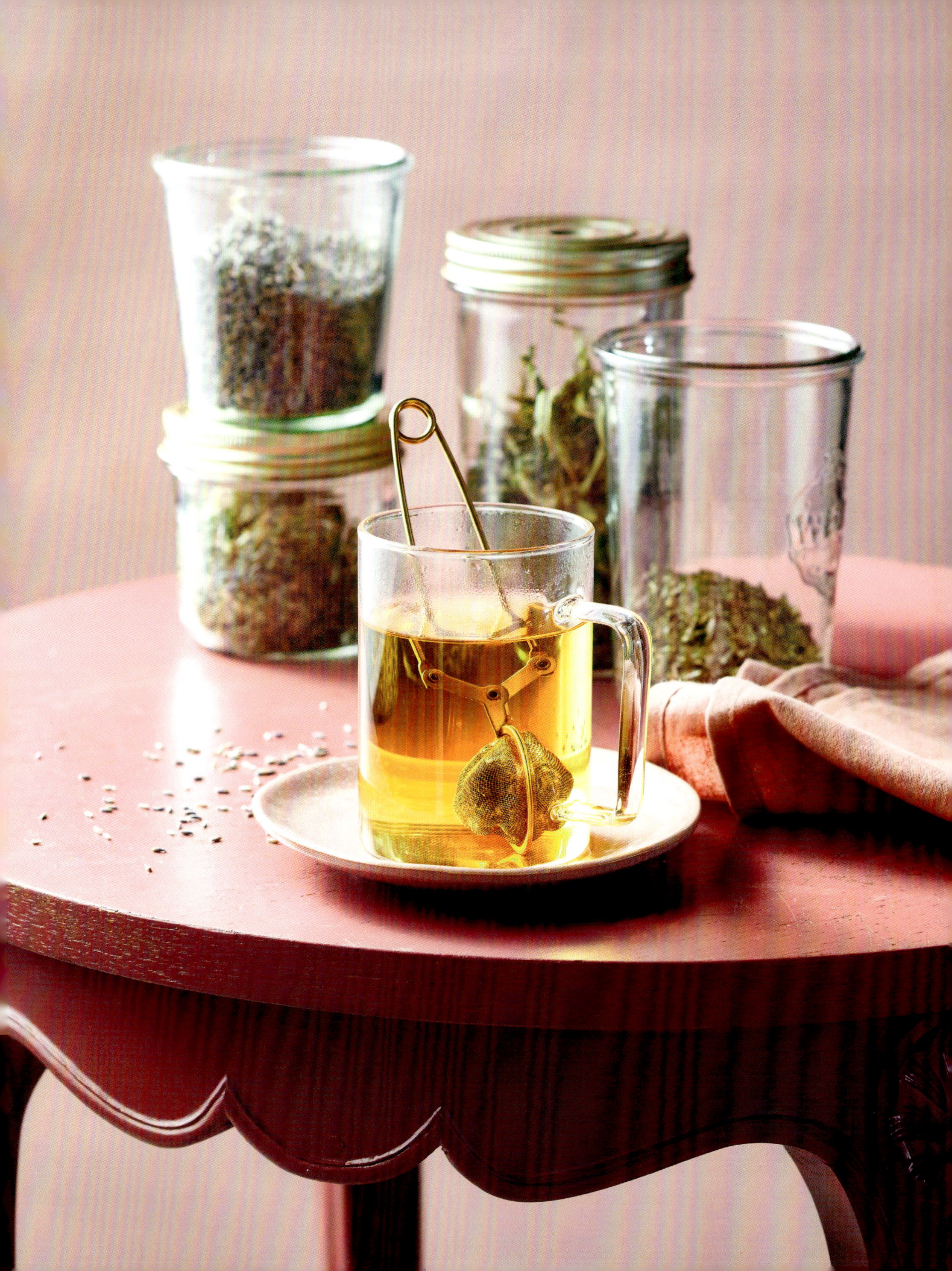

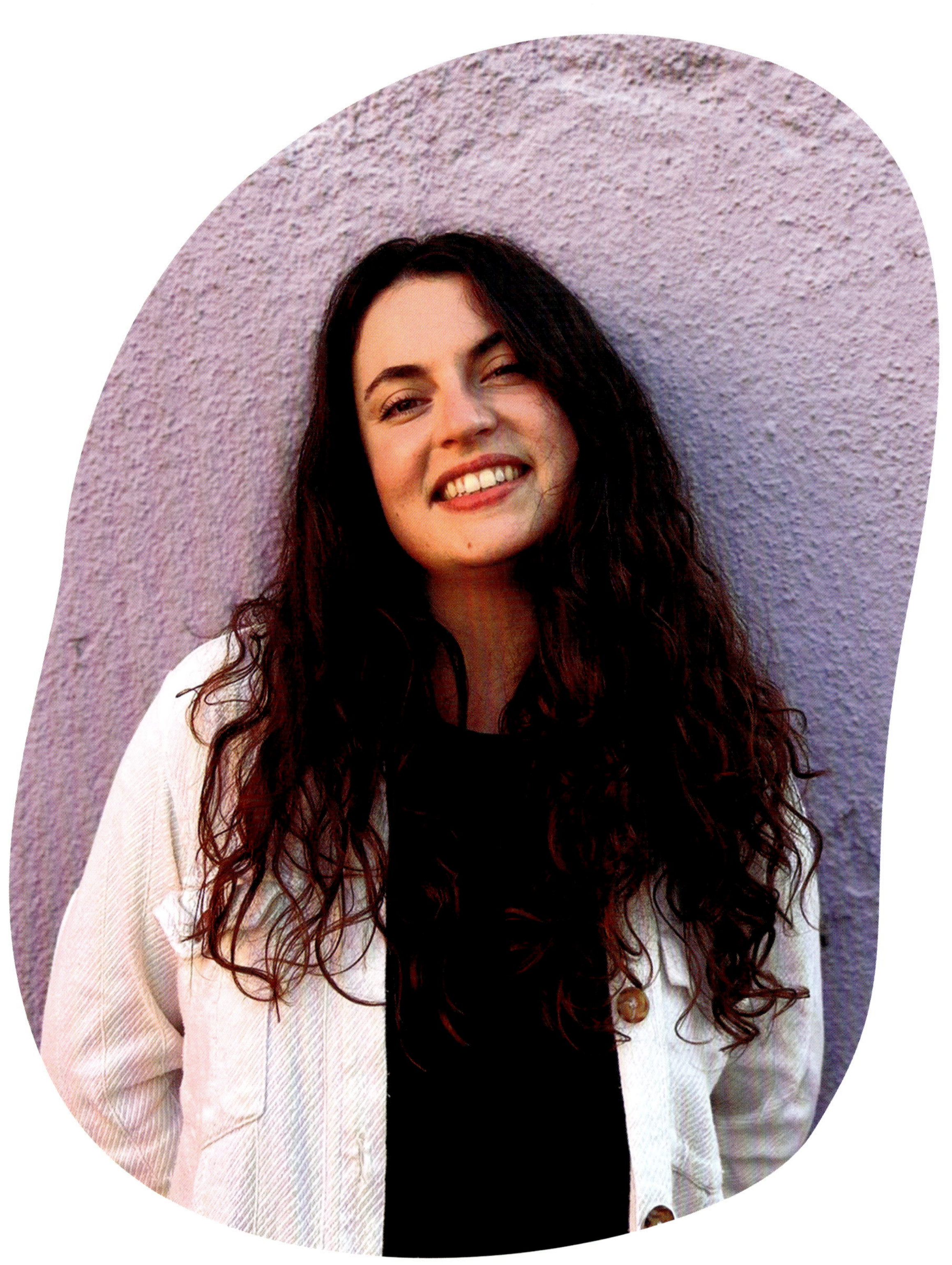

PREFACE

I know what some of you are thinking: Am I honestly writing a book about menopause at the age of twenty-eight? It may seem somewhat unusual—I'll admit that—but although I have yet to experience menopause myself, it is something that will affect every woman at some point. I have also seen firsthand in the lives of my patients and loved ones just how overwhelming it can be. We don't talk about it very much—it's almost taboo—but this is a season in a woman's life when she will face any number of challenges and, at the same time, the very real feeling that no one is able to understand what she is going through.

The silence surrounding menopause is a reflection of a broader reality, which is that the space our society allows women to occupy seems to shrink as they get older. Once a woman turns fifty, her life is supposed to stop and she is meant to make herself as invisible as possible—to disappear—when in reality this is the very moment to celebrate her strength, experience, and resilience. I believe there is something to relish about every chapter in life, and menopause is no exception!

This book is also the fruit of my work as a naturopath. Most of the women I see are going through menopause and come to their appointments with a variety of concerns: hot flashes, sleeping problems, weight gain, vaginal dryness, low energy, etc. We then work together to determine what is causing these symptoms [micronutrient deficiencies, unbalanced gut flora (dysbiosis), hormone imbalance] in order to alleviate them. Naturopathic medicine helps restore balance to the body so that patients can feel well physically and mentally. With that in mind, in this book I wanted to give you the tools to effectively manage menopause through what you eat and pair them with naturopathic strategies (physical activity, stress management, herbal medicine) that will serve you during menopause and well beyond it.

Think of this book as my way of telling you that you are not alone and that you are strong—regardless of your age. In these pages you'll find advice for relieving menopause symptoms through food and taking care of your health while preserving what is most important: the joy of eating. Because yes, it is possible to do something good for yourself and still savor every bite.

Hélène Mailleux

Understanding Menopause

Menopause is a natural physiological process that affects all women. It is the result of a series of hormonal changes that mark the end of a woman's reproductive years. As progesterone and estrogen levels drop, the ovaries gradually stop releasing eggs and the menstrual cycle stops.

PERIMENOPAUSE, PREMENOPAUSE, AND MENOPAUSE

Premenopause refers to all of the physical and mental changes that take place before the onset of **menopause**. **Perimenopause** is the period of time before and after your final menstrual cycle. This phase may last several years and includes the year leading up to your last period. When you have not menstruated for twelve consecutive months, perimenopause is over and you have reached menopause.

To best understand menopause, we have to look at the ovarian cycle. This cycle is governed by the follicles located in the ovaries and is divided into the following stages:

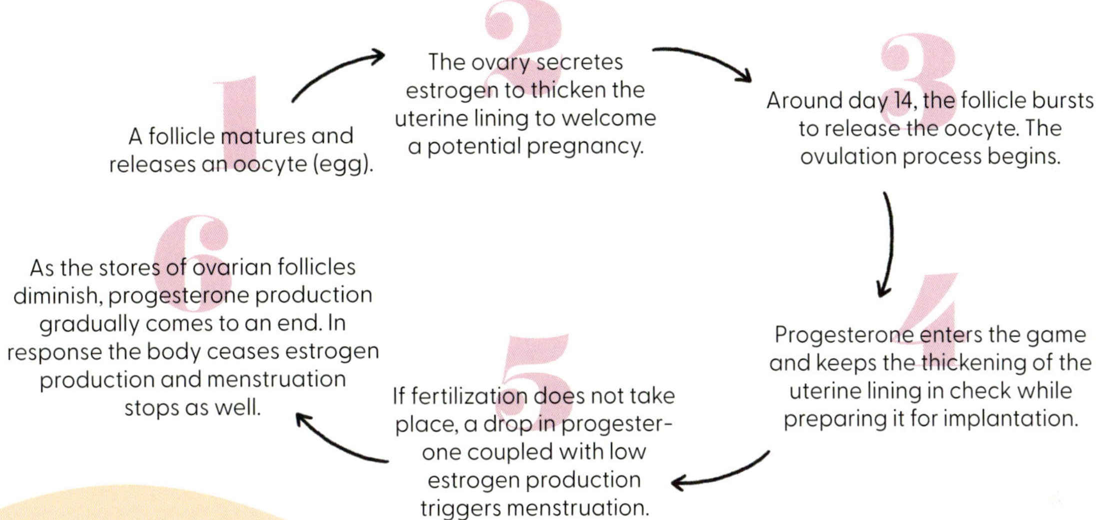

The taboo of menopause

Unfortunately, menopause is still somewhat of a taboo subject, particularly in a society where a woman's worth is often tied to her age and ability to bear children. It is also not something many women look forward to because it can be such a lonely time when many women are ashamed of what is happening to them. This pushes them to keep quiet instead of asking questions to understand what is going on in their bodies.

Menopause is generally believed to be the end of some part of a woman's life. Yet in other cultures and traditional Chinese medicine, the end of menstruation is known as the "second spring"—not an end, then, but a time of renewal and the beginning of a new season in life.

This is a period of transition that can absolutely be enjoyed and made easier with lifestyle changes that complement medical care. For women who suffer from premenstrual syndrome, endometriosis, adenomyosis, and other problems linked to menstruation, menopause can also be a synonym for liberation, relief, and peace.

Menopause is a chance to rethink your habits and create new ones that will help you transition smoothly into this stage of life. The goal of this book is to approach menopause through food. Adding the essential nutrients and micronutrients you'll find in these recipes to your plate each day will equip you to manage a variety of symptoms.

MENOPAUSE SYMPTOMS

Menopause has many symptoms that may appear earlier or later depending on the person. Here are some of them:

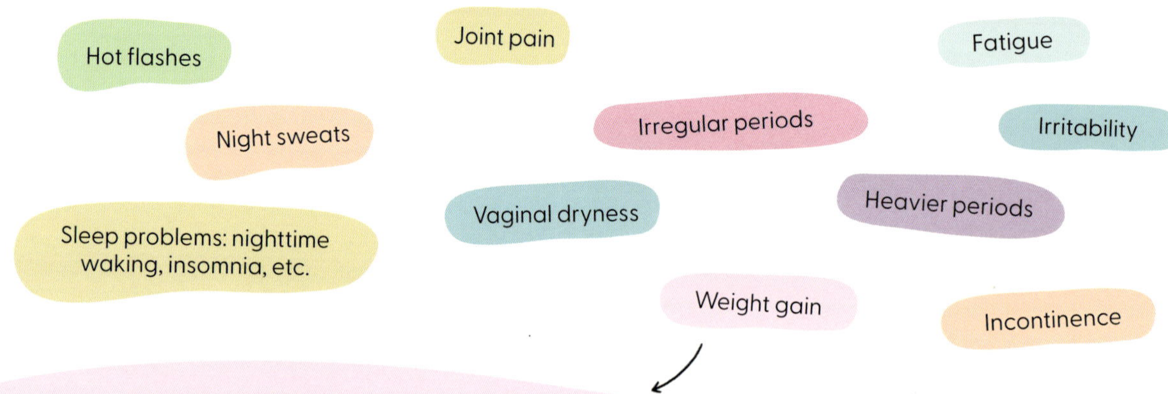

What you should know about weight gain

An initial drop in hormone levels is often observed around the age of forty: This is what is known as perimenopause. The symptoms are identical to those of premenopause, but are usually milder. To cope with this hormone depletion, the body initiates a completely natural and healthy process: weight gain.

Yes, you read that right. Adipose tissue (fat) can bridge this hormonal gap by contributing to estrogen production. Many of my patients and other women I know resist this weight gain by trying as hard as they can to restrict their food intake, increase their physical activity, and eliminate certain foods from their diet. They end up falling into a vicious cycle in which their menopause symptoms actually become more pronounced. If we allow those pounds onto our bodies, this surplus adipose tissue reduces the drop in our hormone levels and symptoms are milder or, in certain women, completely absent.

It's important to keep in mind that there may be other factors contributing to weight gain that are not related to menopause. For example, I often observe that women who are having trouble managing weight gain have reduced their consumption of plant and animal proteins and tend to have a sedentary lifestyle.

Menopause can also cause or exacerbate health issues that are linked to hormonal changes like osteoporosis, cardiovascular disease, diabetes, depression, and bladder/urinary tract issues.

In this book, I'll guide you through all kinds of recipes created specifically for menopause symptoms and their related risks. Every one of these recipes is anti-inflammatory and designed to promote hormonal balance. You'll learn about the key nutrients and micronutrients for a healthy menopause and enjoy eating at the same time.

MANAGING STRESS DURING MENOPAUSE

Hormonal fluctuations during menopause can affect the nervous system, which for some women will mean an increased sensitivity to stress. The symptoms themselves (hot flashes, sleep problems, mood swings) can also contribute to this stress.

Managing stress needs to be high priority during this stage of your life especially. Here are a few tips to make it easier.

Manage your time and commitments

Don't be afraid to take time for yourself and say no to commitments that are not important. Knowing what helps you unwind and find rest is key. It doesn't matter what this looks like for you: It might be a walk outdoors, crafting, gardening, quality time with loved ones, reading, or time spent cooking. Avoiding overload and giving yourself time devoted to some kind of relaxing activity will help reduce stress.

Eat a well-balanced and varied diet

This is what this book is all about. A healthy diet helps reduce stress during menopause whereas certain foods, like those high in sugar and saturated fat, can make symptoms worse. Eating nutritious foods that are rich in micronutrients is a better approach.

Seek out social support

This is so important during menopause. As I mentioned earlier, it can still sometimes feel like a taboo subject. Be proactive and share your concerns, your experiences, your challenges, and your successes with the people around you. The simple act of talking about what you might be feeling will help relieve stress and keep you from feeling like you're totally alone during this time of transition.

Cardiac coherence breathing

This practice relieves anxiety and tension in the body to promote both physical and mental relaxation as well as general well-being. It is an excellent tool for stress management, synchronizing your heartbeat with your breath, dealing with difficult emotions, and can even improve digestion.

Belly breathing—the technique used to stimulate cardiac coherence—stimulates the vagus nerve. The vagus nerve is the major relaxation nerve and influences all of the digestive organs as well. Stimulating this nerve activates the parasympathetic nervous system, which is responsible for digestion. When we are under stress, our stress hormones actually inhibit the parasympathetic nervous system and put us on alert by triggering the sympathetic nervous system.

The 3-6-5 method for practicing cardiac coherence

3 **times a day: morning, noon, and evening**

6 **breaths per minute**

5 **minutes each time**

Breathe in through your nose for **5 seconds**, allowing air to fill your belly. Exhale through your mouth for **5 seconds**, contracting your abdominal muscles. Do this for **5 minutes**.

Count your inhalations and exhalations or download a breathing application on your phone to help.

Maintain regular physical activity

Exercise and movement reduce stress by releasing endorphins, which are feel-good hormones that improve your mood. When we talk about physical activity, we have a tendency to think of physically intense or competitive activities. This is why I prefer the term "movement" which hints at a gentler approach. Choose an activity that you enjoy so you can practice it regularly and find pleasure in it.

MOVEMENT AND PHYSICAL ACTIVITY DURING MENOPAUSE

Being sedentary makes us sick—all of the scientific studies agree on this. It is a major risk factor for cardiovascular disease, bone density loss, weight gain, obesity, and metabolic disorders. Here are some concrete ways to (re)incorporate regular physical activity into your life to make menopause less challenging.

The benefits of physical activity during menopause

Fewer hot flashes and vasomotor symptoms thanks to improved body temperature regulation.

Weight management and metabolism: Physical activity makes it easier to maintain a healthy weight and metabolism, which means it can also help you manage the weight gain associated with menopause.

Stronger bones: Resistance and weight-bearing exercises in particular help maintain bone density and reduce the risk of osteoporosis.

Improved mood and mental well-being: Physical activity stimulates the release of endorphins, the feel-good hormones, which helps reduce stress, anxiety, and the symptoms of depression associated with menopause.

What kind of physical activity should I choose?

I recommend three kinds of physical activity during menopause. Let yourself try whatever piques your interest as you learn about and discover new things along the way:

1. **Cardio exercises** like power walking, running, swimming, and bicycling are excellent ways to strengthen the heart and improve endurance.

2. **Strength training** with free weights, resistance bands, and weight-bearing exercises helps maintain muscle mass and keep bones strong.

3. **Balance and stretching exercises** like yoga, Pilates, and tai chi help develop flexibility, balance, and improve posture as well as your response to everyday stress.

LIMITING EXPOSURE TO ENDOCRINE DISRUPTORS

The endocrine system regulates hormone production and release in the body and endocrine disruptors are chemicals that can interfere with how it functions. These substances cause problems by mimicking, blocking, or altering the action of your natural hormones.

Several studies have examined the link between exposure to endocrine disruptors and menopause symptoms like hot flashes, joint pain, and vaginal dryness.

A study published in *Environmental Health Perspectives*[1] revealed that women exposed to high levels of endocrine disruptors like phthalates and bisphenols were more likely to suffer from hot flashes and night sweats. In addition, these chemical compounds have been found to affect the health of vaginal tissues and make vaginal dryness worse. These substances—which are found in most traditional cosmetic products, perfumes, and plastic packaging for food and nonfood items—can disrupt hormonal balance and exacerbate the vasomotor symptoms associated with menopause.

Other research[2] has shown that the chemicals present in plastics and pesticides may contribute to chronic inflammation and joint pain. Another study published in *Environmental Research* showed a link between pesticide exposure and an increased risk of joint pain in menopausal women.

My tips for limiting exposure to endocrine disruptors in daily life

1

Change your skincare and makeup routine

Industrial cosmetics are full of endocrine disruptors. Here's how they'll appear on a list of ingredients (these are called their INCI names): butylparaben, propylparaben, methylparaben, ethylparaben, diethyl phthalate, phthalic acid, BHA, triclosan, resorcinol, methylchloroisothiazolinone, ethylhexyl methoxycinnamate, etc. There are plenty of alternative brands that you can use in place of traditional products.

2

Use environmentally friendly cleaning products

Many conventional cleaning products contain endocrine disruptors. Try to use eco-certified products or natural solutions like white vinegar, baking soda, castile soap, etc.

3

Avoid plastics containing bisphenol A (BPA)

These are often found in plastic packaging for food and nonfood items. As often as possible, choose containers made of glass, stainless steel, or another BPA-free material for storing food.

[1] https://www.sciencedirect.com/science/article/pii/S0048969721072880.

[2] https://ehp.niehs.nih.gov/doi/10.1289/isee.2021.P-441.

4

Avoid using aluminum utensils and containers

Use stainless steel for cooking whenever possible. Use glass containers for storing food. Beeswax wrap, a food wrap made out of organic beeswax and organic cotton, is another option (just make sure it's GOTS and OEKO-TEX 100 certified).

6

Eat organic

The pesticides used in conventional agriculture may contain endocrine disruptors. As much as possible, eat organic foods to reduce your exposure to pesticides.

5

Reduce your exposure to chemicals in the home

Some chemicals found in furniture, floor treatments, and paint can also be endocrine disruptors. Choose products that do not contain toxins and regularly air out your home to reduce exposure.

NATUROPATHIC SUPPORT DURING MENOPAUSE

A large portion of my work as a naturopath involves helping women deal with the challenges of menopause. This phase in life can be accompanied by a range of troublesome symptoms that you, my reader, may also be dealing with in your daily life.

Naturopathy offers a holistic, personalized wellness approach to help you move through this season comfortably and peacefully. Together, you and your naturopath can create a plan that will respond to your individual needs while keeping in mind your medical history, symptoms, and lifestyle.

Natural treatment methods can act as a complement to your regular medical care to help balance your hormones. Combining these approaches with healthy and tasty recipes offers even greater support for your hormonal well-being and will ease your transition through menopause.

Building a Healthy Plate during Menopause

Menopause through Diet

Menopause is much more than the end of your period—it's an opportunity to rethink your relationship with food and revitalize your body with healthy snacks and meals. I have put together a selection of recipes to help you do just that.

Instead of cutting out certain foods altogether, the naturopathic approach adds raw and living foods to your diet to fill you up with vitamins, minerals, and essential nutrients in order to boost your energy levels, immune system, and hormonal balance.

With this in mind, we need to highlight a few of these key nutrients: protein, fiber, calcium, vitamins D and K, omega-3, and zinc. Foods containing these nutrients help the body synthesize hormones to cope with the drop in estrogen and progesterone that is responsible for menopause symptoms.

As you read through this book, you'll discover delicious and creative ways to add these important ingredients to your own plate. Whether you're looking for comfort food, energizing smoothies, or simple everyday meals, I've made sure that each recipe not only tastes amazing but is also beneficial for your overall health.

WHAT KINDS OF FOODS SHOULD I BE PUTTING ON MY PLATE?

Make sure you're getting enough protein

Including the right amount of protein in your diet is important for muscle and bone health, weight management, and hormone regulation. During menopause, eating protein promotes optimal body composition and helps preserve muscle mass and strength. Protein is also critical for bone health because it provides the amino acids that are necessary for bone tissue formation and repair.

Managing your weight can become difficult during menopause because of the metabolic and hormonal changes at work in the body. Getting enough protein stabilizes blood sugar, increases satiety, and also promotes neurotransmitter production. Neurotransmitters are chemical messengers that influence our mood, motivation, sleep, and more.

How much protein should I be eating?

1 or 2 grams for every kilogram you weigh (a kilogram is equal to 2.2 pounds)

Example: A woman who weighs 75 kg (165 lbs) needs:
75 × 1 = 75 g
to
75 × 2 = 150 g
(5.3 ounces) of protein spread out over the day.

Protein content

1 egg	6 g of protein
3.5oz (100 g) fromage blanc (sheep or goat's milk)	7 g of protein
3.5 oz (100 g) skyr yogurt (sheep or goat's milk)	10 g of protein
3.5 oz (100 g) fatty fish (sardine, mackerel, herring, salmon, etc.)	13 g of protein
3.5 oz (100 g) oilseeds	15 g of protein
3.5 oz (100 g) white meat (chicken, turkey)	20 g of protein
3.5 oz (100 g) cheese	20 g of protein

You will find a more detailed list of foods on page 38.

Be careful not to confuse the portion size of a particular food with the actual amount of protein you are getting. For example, 100 grams of chicken, lentils, or tofu does not contain 100 grams of protein. In reality, 100 grams of chicken contains 20 to 23 grams of protein, whereas 100 grams of cooked lentils contains 9 grams. All foods are made up of water, fiber, lipids, and other nutrients. This reduces the amount of protein they contain. It is therefore essential to get protein from a variety of different foods to make sure your body is getting what it needs.

Eat more fiber

Fiber plays an important role in maintaining digestive health: It helps keep bowel movements regular, prevents constipation, and promotes healthy gut bacteria (this is because fiber contains prebiotics that nourish the probiotics in the intestines). Hormonal fluctuations during menopause can slow digestion, and fiber is especially important during this time.

Fiber can also regulate blood sugar levels and increase feelings of satiety, which can be useful if you are trying to manage your weight. If you haven't already, take a look at "What you should know about weight gain" (page 10).

Soluble fiber

Fiber helps lower the glycemic index (GI) of the foods we eat. Soluble fiber in particular slows down digestion and carbohydrate absorption in the intestine. It is found in foods like oats, legumes, apples, and citrus fruits.

When in contact with water, soluble fiber dissolves to form a gel-like substance that slows the passage of food through the digestive system and the absorption of glucose into the blood. This helps avoid rapid blood glucose spikes after a meal. Instead of a steep and elevated increase of blood glucose, the rise in glucose will be slower and more moderate. Stable levels of blood glucose prevent sugar crashes and cravings.

Menopause is associated with an increased risk of cardiovascular disease because of the changes to a woman's estrogen levels. Fiber in general—and soluble fiber in particular—can help reduce levels of LDL cholesterol (the "bad" cholesterol) and improve heart health.

Insoluble fiber

Although insoluble fiber does not dissolve in water, it does add bulk to the stool and accelerates bowel transit time. This can contribute to slower carbohydrate absorption because foods pass more quickly through the digestive tract and certain nutrients may have less time to be absorbed. Thanks to its effects on hormonal regulation, fiber also plays an indirect role in reducing menopause symptoms like hot flashes and night sweats.

Blood glucose curve after eating:

Foods with elevated GI (> 70)

Foods with moderate GI (> 55 and < 70).

Low IG (< 55)

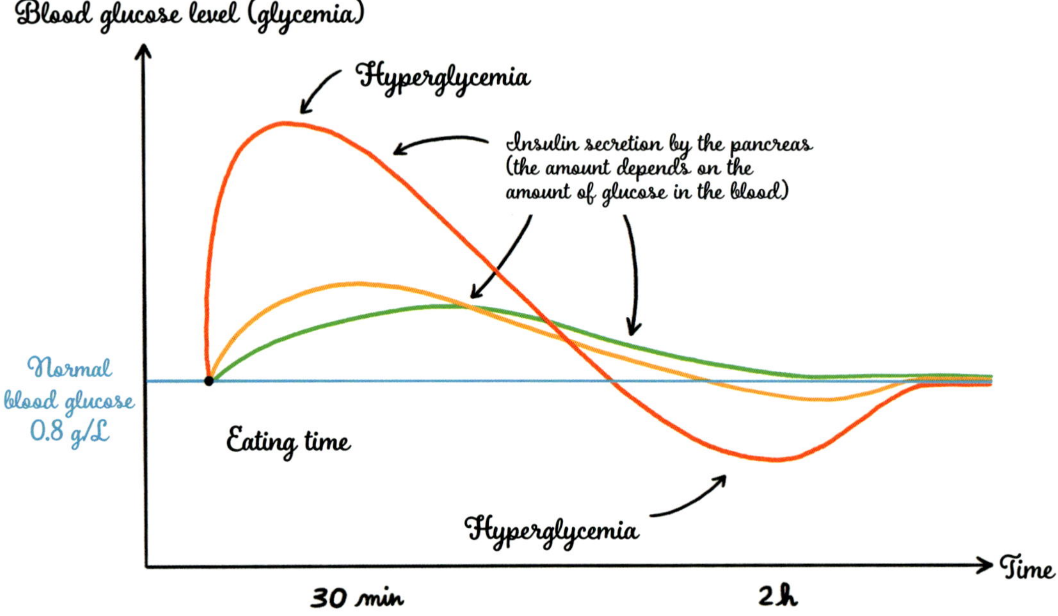

Which foods contain fiber?

Soluble fiber

This dissolves in water to form a gel-like substance that helps slow down digestion and carbohydrate absorption. It helps reduce cholesterol and regulates blood sugar levels.

Fruits

Apples, citrus (oranges, grapefruit), strawberries, pears, peaches, prunes, nectarines

Soaked legumes*

Beans (white, red, black, cranberry, pinto, mung, adzuki, soy, flageolet, fava), lentils (green, brown, black, coral), chickpeas, split peas, yellow peas

Vegetables

Carrots, zucchini, broccoli, Brussels sprouts, sweet potatoes

Grains and seeds

Oat and oat bran, barley, rye, quinoa

Other

Chia seeds, flaxseed, psyllium

*Soaking legumes destroys phytic acid, an antinutrient that is naturally present in grains, dried legumes, seeds, and oilseeds. It is stored in the seed coat to help the seed germinate and grow. Unfortunately, when we consume it, phytic acid blocks certain micronutrients from being absorbed.

Insoluble fiber

This does not dissolve in water and adds bulk to the stool, which in turn speeds up bowel transit time and prevents constipation.

Fruits

Apples (with the skin), bananas, grapes, raspberries, kiwis

Grains

Whole wheat and wheat bran (ancient varieties*), whole wheat bread (preferably sourdough**), brown rice, barley, millet, bulgur

Seeds

Chia seeds, flaxseed

Vegetables

Green beans, cabbage (red, green), cauliflower, spinach, eggplant, Brussels sprouts

Soaked legumes

Beans (white, red, black, cranberry, pinto, mung, adzuki, soy, flageolet, fava), lentils (green, brown, black, coral), chickpeas

*Ancient grain varieties are not genetically modified and therefore contain less gluten. This makes them easier to digest.

**Yeast predigests the gluten and destroys phytic acid, which makes the bread easier to digest.

Calcium, vitamins D and K, magnesium, zinc, and omega-3s

Calcium

Estrogen is essential for maintaining bone density because it inhibits bone resorption, which is a natural process that breaks down bone and releases minerals into the blood. The drop in estrogen levels during menopause increases your risk of bone density loss and osteoporosis.

Calcium is crucial for solid bone structure, preventing fractures and teeth problems, healthy muscle function, nervous system communication, and blood pressure regulation. It also plays a role in a number of metabolic processes related to weight management. *For more information, see "Nutrition Close-Up" on page 63.*

Vitamins D and K

Vitamin D is essential for good calcium absorption, which is important during menopause for maintaining bone density and preventing osteoporosis. Without vitamin D, adequate levels of calcium will be unable to do anything for your body. Vitamin D also improves muscle function, strengthens the immune system, and helps regulate mood.

Vitamin K works together with vitamin D by directing calcium in the blood to the bones. It also plays a role in blood clotting and helps prevent calcification in the arteries. *For more information, see "Nutrition Close-Up" on page 64.*

Zinc

The body's zinc needs increase during menopause as a result of hormonal fluctuations. This mineral plays a role in progesterone production and contributes to bone health by promoting bone formation and density. Zinc also helps the body synthesize collagen to keep hair and nails healthy and strong. Zinc strengthens the immune system and supports cognitive function, concentration, and memory. *For more information, see "Nutrition Close-Up" on page 29.*

Magnesium

Magnesium is crucial for bone health because it helps convert vitamin D to its active form for better calcium absorption. It is important for muscle function and can ease the cramps and pains that are frequent during menopause. Magnesium also regulates neurotransmitters—which affect mood and nerve signal transmission—all while playing an essential role in energy production and metabolism regulation. *For more information, see "Nutrition Close-Up" on page 30.*

Omega-3s

The essential fatty acids we call omega-3s are a boost for your cardiovascular health thanks to their anti-inflammatory and antithrombotic properties. Omega-3s reduce inflammation, improve vascular function, and regulate blood lipids to lower the risk of heart disease. They also promote bone density—reducing the risk of osteoporosis—and support mental wellness by regulating mood and reducing symptoms of depression and anxiety.

During menopause, omega-3s' anti-inflammatory properties help reduce chronic inflammation, joint pain, and hot flashes to foster your overall well-being. *For more information, see "Nutrition Close-Up" on page 127.*

THE IMPORTANCE OF CHEWING AND HYDRATION

Chewing

Digestion begins in the mouth with proper chewing. Chewing correctly mixes your food with salivary enzymes and begins the process of breaking down carbohydrates. This gives your digestive enzymes and intestines less work to do. If you don't chew enough, your stomach has to work harder and use more energy. Chewing well also releases nutrients, reduces the likelihood of digestive issues, and helps regulate hunger and satiety to promote better weight management. Taking the time to chew improves digestion and allows you to truly relish whatever you happen to be eating.

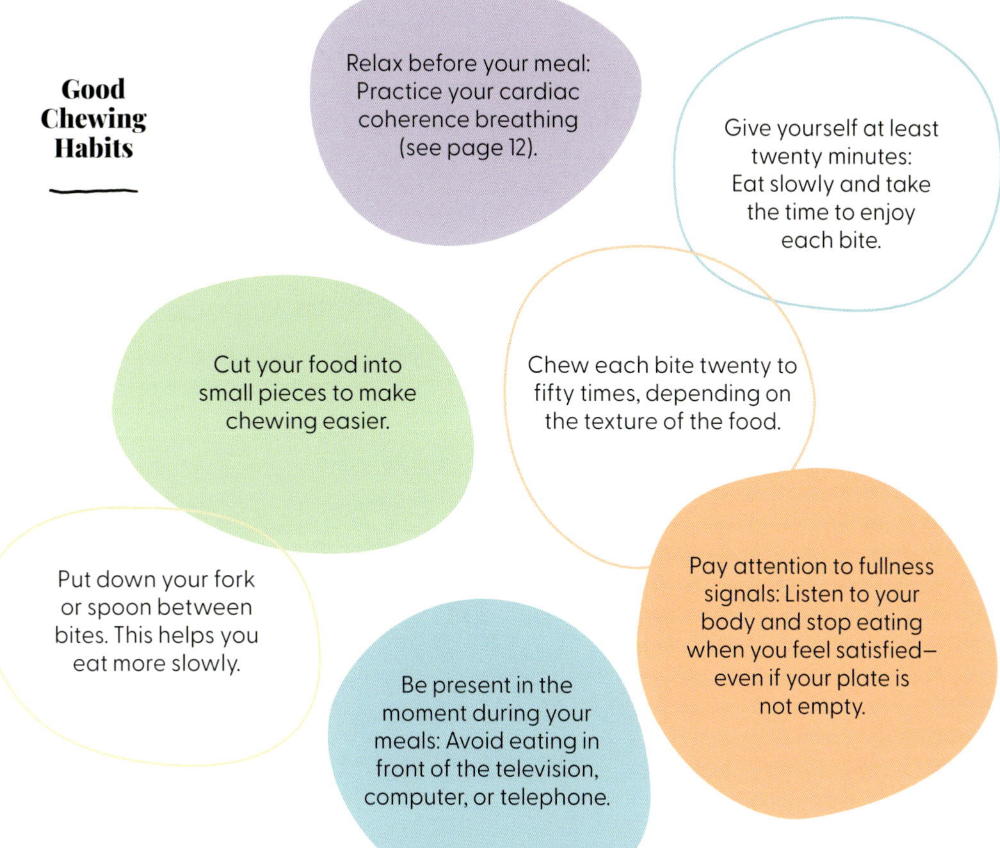

Hydration

Drinking enough water is vital for many of the body's most important processes including body temperature regulation, nutrient transport, waste elimination, joint lubrication, organ protection, and cognitive function. You need to be drinking plenty of water throughout the day to stay hydrated and support your body.

Tips for optimal hydration

Start and finish your day with a glass of water.

Set an alarm on your telephone to go off every hour or use a water reminder app.

Invest in a water bottle you can take with you everywhere.

For every cup of coffee, black tea, or herbal tea, drink 1 glass of water.

Monitor the color of your urine throughout the day.

Very good | Good | OK | Slightly dehydrated | Dehydrated | Very dehydrated | Severely dehydrated

Water needs vary from one person to another. Here's how to calculate the amount you should be drinking every day:

Daily water intake = 0.03 × weight in kg (a kilogram is equal to 2.2 pounds) or, alternatively, 0.014 × your weight in pounds.

For example, a woman who weighs 165 pounds (75 kg) needs 0.03 × 75 = 2.25 liters of water per day or, alternatively, needs 0.014 × 165 = 2.25 liters of water per day

You can also use this checklist to remember when to drink water throughout the day. I have found this tool very helpful for my patients!

Drink 11 glasses of water (8.5 fluid ounces [25 cl] each)

12
3
6
9
1 glass of water when you wake up
1 glass of water before breakfast
2 glasses of water in the morning
1 glass of water before lunch
2 glasses of water in the afternoon
1 glass of water before dinner
2 glasses of water in the evening
1 glass of water 30 minutes before bed

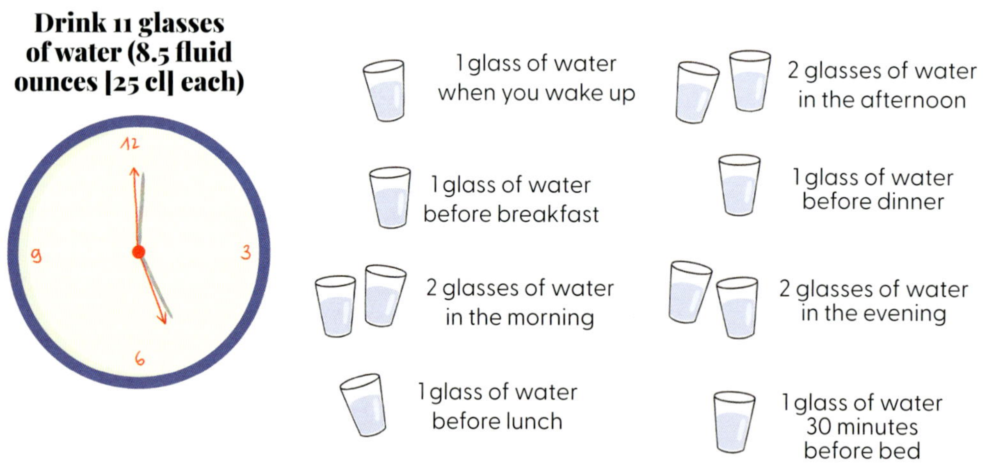

WHAT EXACTLY SHOULD I BE PUTTING ON MY PLATE?

To make sure you're getting the nutrients you need, you'll have to include a variety of foods to meet your macronutrient, micronutrient, and fiber needs. This is what an ideal plate looks like:

50 percent vegetables (raw and cooked)

Vegetables provide an abundance of vitamins, fiber, and minerals that are essential for optimal health. The goal is to combine a variety of raw and cooked vegetables to maximize these nutritional benefits. Raw vegetables tend to preserve more of their vitamins and enzymes, but everything depends on your digestive tolerance. If you can't eat raw vegetables, drink fresh-pressed vegetable juice instead. Juices will not contain the fiber found in raw vegetables and are easy for sensitive stomachs to digest. Cooked vegetables are also easier to digest and offer different flavor possibilities.

25 percent protein

Protein is essential for tissue construction and repair, as well as healthy immune system function. Choose protein sources like chicken, turkey, fish, eggs, tofu, and legumes. Vary your protein sources to make sure you're getting all of the essential amino acids you need.

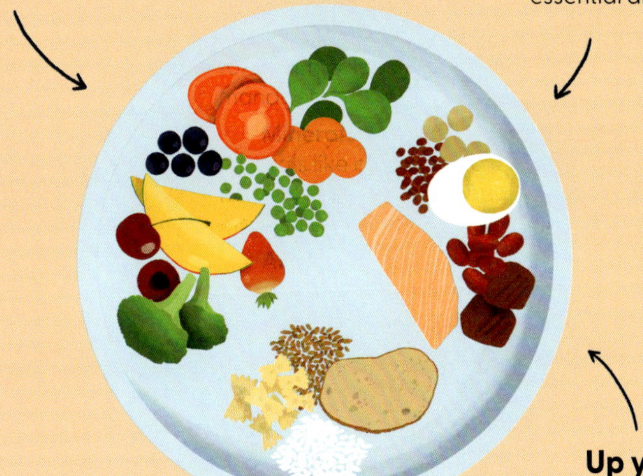

Up your fats

You need fat on your plate for healthy skin, balanced hormones, and to absorb fat-soluble vitamins. Choose healthy fats like avocados, nuts, seeds, unrefined plant oils (olive oil, canola oil, flaxseed oil), and small fatty fish rich in omega-3s.

25 percent carbohydrates

Carbohydrates provide energy. Opt for carbohydrates with a low glycemic index like whole grains, legumes, tubers, and root vegetables. These release energy over a longer period of time and are rich in fiber, which helps you feel full and stabilizes blood sugar levels.

NUTRITION CLOSE-UP

Don't Skimp on Spices

Spices are an effective, natural way to support your health during menopause and they also add something special to your recipes. The list below will help you choose spices to cook with when you are experiencing symptoms:

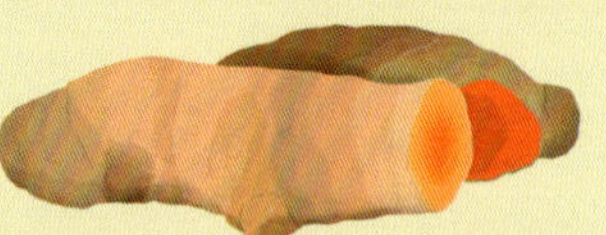

Hot Flashes

• Sage • Cinnamon •
• Turmeric • Ginger •

These spices help regulate body temperature and reduce the intensity and frequency of hot flashes.

Inflammation

• Turmeric • Ginger •
• Black pepper • Cinnamon •

These anti-inflammatory spices fight chronic inflammation from the inside to relieve pain and swelling in muscles and joints. Always pair turmeric with ginger to optimize its effects—the curcumin in turmeric is activated by the gingerol in ginger.

Mood and Mental Health

• Saffron • Turmeric •
• Cardamom • Cinnamon •

These spices are adaptogens, which means they can help regulate stress, improve mood, and promote a sense of mental well-being.

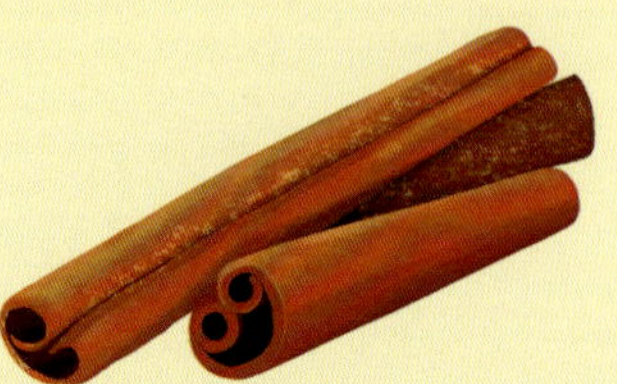

Digestion

• Ginger • Cardamom •
• Cinnamon • Cumin •

These digestive spices have carminative properties that can relieve gastrointestinal problems like bloating, gas, and other digestive issues.

Plants and Their Soothing Properties

NUTRITION CLOSE-UP

Whether you're cooking with them or simply making a cup of tea, aromatic herbs offer a number of benefits during menopause. You don't need to search far and wide, either—our gardens are full of helpful plants!

Rosemary

Rosemary has antioxidant and anti-inflammatory properties that relieve hot flashes, improve blood circulation, and strengthen immunity. It also promotes digestion and can help lower blood sugar levels.

Thyme

Thyme is an invigorating antimicrobial plant that wards off fatigue and anxiety and strengthens immunity. It is also effective against inflammation and can help combat urinary tract infections.

Dill

Dill has anti-inflammatory and antimicrobial properties as well as digestive benefits. It can be used to fight infections and is also an antioxidant.

Oregano

Oregano is rich in antioxidant and antimicrobial compounds, strengthens the immune system, reduces inflammation, and improves digestion.

Basil

Basil is an antioxidant with anti-inflammatory and antimicrobial properties that protect cells, reduce inflammation, and fight infections. It is also good for digestion and can improve mood.

Chives

Chives are rich in vitamins and antioxidants which strengthen the immune system and protect cells. They also have anti-inflammatory and digestive benefits.

Cilantro

Cilantro is known for its cell-protecting powers as an antioxidant as well as its anti-inflammatory and antimicrobial properties. This herb reduces inflammation and fights infection. It is also good for digestion and reducing toxicity in the body.

Tarragon

Tarragon is an antioxidant with anti-inflammatory and antimicrobial properties that strengthen cells, support digestion, and reduce blood sugar levels.

Parsley

Parsley is rich in vitamins and antioxidants that strengthen the immune system, protect cells, and support bone health. It also has anti-inflammatory and diuretic properties that reduce inflammation and eliminate toxins from the body.

Fennel

Fennel leaves and seeds are antioxidants that possess a variety of benefits including cell protection, reduced inflammation, and improved digestion. They are also rich in fiber, vitamins, and minerals that promote general well-being and support the immune system.

Sprouted Seeds

Sprouted seeds are rich in vitamins, minerals, and enzymes to strengthen the immune system and improve digestion. They also offer antioxidant benefits that protect cells.

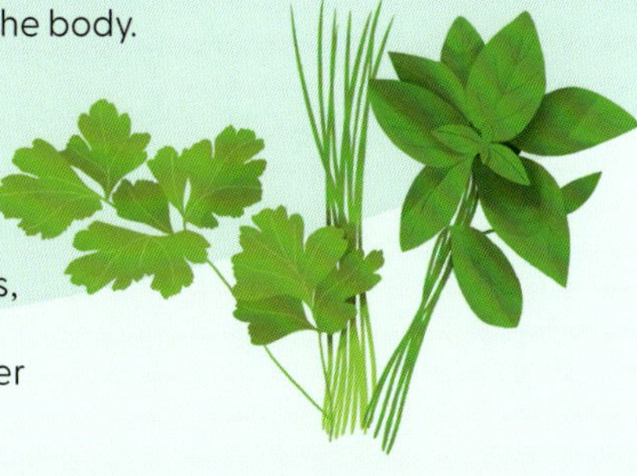

MENOPAUSE KITCHEN STAPLES

These ingredients can be found in organic grocery stores, Asian markets, and online.

Fresh Produce

- Sprouted seeds
- Kimchi
- Sheep's milk
- Goat's milk
- Soy milk
- Lacto-fermented vegetables
- Fresh yeast
- Parmesan
- Firm tofu
- Lacto-fermented tofu
- Silken tofu

Savory Recipes

- Canned cod liver
- Canned small fatty fish, bone-in
- Lupine flour
- Whole-grain rice flour
- Buckwheat flour
- High-gluten or whole wheat flours
- Fava beans
- Fleur de sel (to replace table salt)
- Flageolet beans
- Ghee (clarified butter that does not contain lactose or casein)
- Adzuki beans
- White beans
- Mung beans
- Black beans
- Pinto beans
- Cranberry beans
- Red beans
- Cold-pressed olive oil
- Omega-3 oils: canola hemp, flaxseed
- Miso
- Rice noodles
- Split peas
- Chickpeas
- Yellow peas
- White rice
- Whole-grain rice
- Soba (buckwheat noodles)
- Soy sauce
- Tamari
- Apple cider vinegar

Sweet Recipes

- Dates
- Gluten-free oats
- Raw honey
- Almond butter
- Tahini
- Maple syrup
- Coconut sugar
- Muscovado sugar

Nuts and Seeds

- Almonds
- Hulled hemp seeds
- Chia seeds
- Flaxseeds
- Hazelnuts
- Cashews
- Walnuts
- Brazil nuts
- Pistachios
- Black and white sesame seeds

Herbs and Spices

- Cinnamon
- Cardamom
- Cilantro
- Turmeric
- Ginger
- Gomasio (a blend of sesame seeds and salt that is another alternative to table salt)
- Parsley
- Sage

Other

- Seaweed (wakame, dulse, royal kombu)
- Natto (in Asian markets)
- Psyllium (check the supplement aisle in organic grocery stores)

WHY YOU SHOULD BE EATING SEASONAL FRUITS AND VEGETABLES

Eating produce that is in season has many nutritional, environmental, and economic benefits.

Better flavor

Seasonal fruits and vegetables—especially if they are locally grown—are picked when they are ripe. This means they offer a more pronounced flavor and just the right texture. There's just nothing like a juicy summer tomato or a crunchy autumn pear!

Higher nutrient content

Fruits and vegetables that are harvested and eaten in season are generally richer in essential nutrients and correspond to the human body's needs in every season. In the winter, the body needs warmth, nutrients, and vitamin C to support the immune system. This makes it the perfect time for winter vegetable soups and citrus. In the summer, the body is calling out for refreshment and hydration and nature offers us water-filled vegetables and fruits such as cucumbers, squash, melons, and tomatoes

Respect for nature's cycle

Eating seasonally puts you in sync with the earth's natural cycle. This promotes a more sustainable local agriculture industry, reduces our dependence on imported food, and helps bolster farming practices that are respectful of the environment.

Better for your budget

Seasonal products are often cheaper because they are available in abundance at harvesttime. This lets you save money without compromising on quality.

More variety in your diet

Every season offers a wide variety of fruits and vegetables, so you can maintain a balanced diet with different kinds of produce all year long. The recipes in this book are made to work in every season. Decide what you're in the mood for and choose from whatever vegetables are available!

Recipes for Hormonal Balance

The hormonal fluctuations of menopause can cause a variety of symptoms like mood swings and a drop in energy. A diet rich in zinc and magnesium helps support natural hormone balance and alleviate these problems. Throughout this book we'll be talking about other essential micronutrients that can make this season easier for you.

Zinc

During menopause, the body's zinc needs may increase because of the hormonal changes and health challenges that are unique to this time in a woman's life. This is why zinc is particularly important during menopause.

Hormonal regulation
Zinc plays a role in regulating thyroid hormones, estrogen, and progesterone production. It can help relieve certain menopause symptoms like hot flashes and night sweats by promoting hormonal stability.

Bone health
With the decrease in estrogen levels, menopausal women are at a greater risk for developing osteoporosis. Zinc contributes to bone formation and mineralization, helping to maintain bone density and prevent bone fragility.

Healthy skin and hair
Menopause can change our skin and hair and cause problems like dryness and hair loss. Zinc is essential for collagen production and tissue repair and helps promote healthy skin and strong hair.

Zinc also supports the immune system by helping fight off infections and promoting an effective immune response. It is also involved in brain function and boosts concentration and memory.

Foods High in Zinc

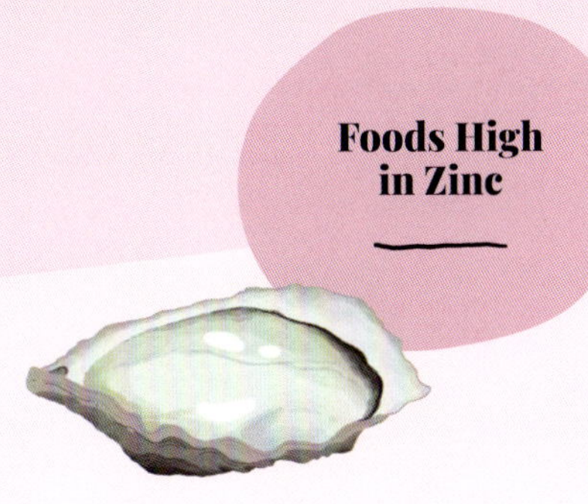

Animal products
Beef, pork, chicken, lamb, turkey, eggs

Seafood and shellfish
Oysters, crab and lobster, mussels, shrimp

Dairy products
Cheese, yogurt, milk
For information about choosing the best dairy products, *see page 108.*

Legumes
Chickpeas, lentils, black beans, white beans, edamame

Nuts and seeds
Pumpkin seeds, sesame seeds, chia seeds, flaxseed, cashews, pine nuts, almonds, Brazil nuts

Vegetables
Spinach, mushrooms (shiitakes especially), asparagus, broccoli

Grains
Quinoa, oats, brown rice, whole-grain sourdough bread, whole wheat pasta

Other
Raw cacao, wheat germ, nutritional yeast

NUTRITION CLOSE-UP

Magnesium

Magnesium is an essential mineral that plays a role in many of the body's functions (see page 154 for more).

Magnesium is vital for bone health because it activates vitamin D, which promotes calcium absorption in the bones. Roughly 60 percent of the body's magnesium is found in the bones.

This mineral is also critical for muscle contraction and relaxation. It helps prevent the frequent cramps and muscle pains that come with menopause.

Magnesium plays a role in nerve signal transmission and is also involved in regulating neurotransmitters, which are chemicals that transmit messages between nerve cells and muscles. Serotonin, a mood booster, is one of those neurotransmitters.

Getting enough magnesium ensures healthy nerve communication and prevents certain neurological problems. Magnesium plays a key role in regulating the body's response to stress. It is also necessary for the production of ATP (the cell's primary energy source) and helps the body maintain stable levels of energy.

Magnesium is crucial for producing and storing energy. The body needs magnesium for over 300 different reactions including fat and carbohydrate metabolism and blood sugar and insulin regulation. In other words, magnesium helps maintain healthy metabolism and manage weight effectively.

Foods High in Magnesium

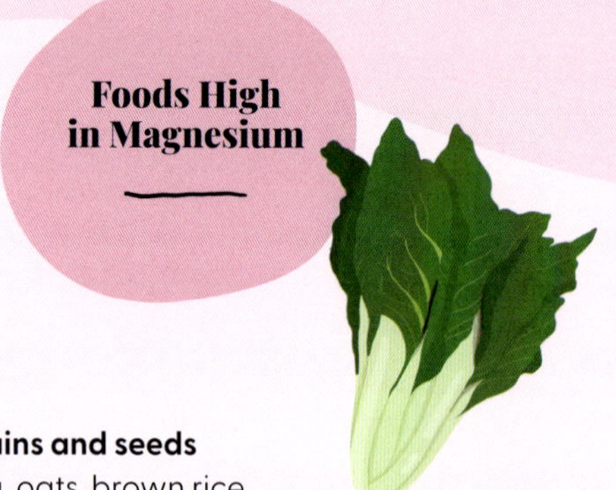

Grains and seeds

Quinoa, oats, brown rice, buckwheat, barley, millet

Green vegetables

Broccoli, kale, cabbage, spinach, Swiss chard, green lettuce, arugula, lamb's lettuce (corn salad)

Fruit

Avocado, banana, figs, raisins, dates, kiwi

Fatty fish

Sardines, mackerel, wild salmon, herring, wild tuna, anchovies

Nuts and seeds

Almonds, pumpkin seeds, sesame seeds, cashews, Brazil nuts, flaxseed, chia seeds, sunflower seeds

Legumes

Black beans, white beans, lentils, chickpeas, edamame

Other

Dark chocolate, tofu, nutritional yeast, wheat germ

Getting enough magnesium during menopause is particularly important for several reasons:

Managing stress and anxiety

Women in menopause often experience stress and anxiety as a result of hormonal fluctuations. Magnesium helps regulate the nervous system by acting as a natural relaxant. It also plays a part in the production of neurotransmitters like serotonin, which promotes feelings of well-being and helps reduce anxiety and stress.

Better sleep

Sleep problems are common during menopause. Magnesium plays a key role in sleep regulation by promoting muscle and nerve relaxation. It can also help improve the quality of your sleep by regulating production of the sleep hormone melatonin.

Bone health

Decreased estrogen levels during menopause can cause bone density loss and increase your risk of osteoporosis. Magnesium is essential for bone formation and calcium absorption to maintain solid, healthy bones.

Blood sugar regulation

Menopause can increase your risk of insulin resistance and type 2 diabetes. Magnesium helps regulate blood sugar through more than 300 different enzyme reactions, including those involved in carbohydrate and fat metabolism. It also improves insulin sensitivity, which helps stabilize sugar levels in the blood.

Fewer hot flashes and night sweats

Thanks to its role in regulating nerve and muscle function, magnesium can help reduce the frequency and intensity of hot flashes and night sweats.

Gluten-Free Veggie and Pumpkin Seed Muffins

Makes 12 muffins
Prep: 15 minutes
Cook: 25 minutes

Fall/Winter Version:

1 small sweet potato

1 carrot

1 small onion

1.75 ounces (50 g) kale

Spring/Summer Version:

1 zucchini

1 carrot

1 small onion

1 red bell pepper

7 ounces (200 g) whole-grain rice flour

2½ teaspoons (11 g) gluten-free baking powder

2 eggs

3.5 fluid ounces (100 ml) plant-based milk

2 tablespoons olive oil

1.75 ounces (50 g) pumpkin seeds

Salt and pepper

RECIPE

Preheat the oven to 350°F (180°C).

Grate, chop, or thinly slice the vegetables. Combine the flour and baking powder. Beat the eggs together with the milk and oil.

Pour the wet mixture over the dry ingredients and stir until combined. Add the vegetables and pumpkin seeds, then season with salt and pepper and gently stir everything together.

Transfer the batter to a muffin tin and bake for 20 to 25 minutes until the muffins are golden brown and the tip of a knife inserted in the center of a muffin comes out clean.

HOW IT HELPS YOUR BODY

Fiber and digestive: Whole-grain rice flour and grated vegetables provide plenty of fiber, which is essential for healthy digestion, blood sugar regulation, and preventing constipation.

Vitamins and minerals: Seasonal vegetables provide a variety of vitamins and minerals. Sweet potatoes and carrots, for instance, are rich in vitamin A and antioxidants that support healthy skin and immunity. Kale and bell peppers also provide vitamin C, which is important for bone health and energy.

Protein: Eggs and pumpkin seeds provide high-quality protein that is essential for maintaining muscle mass. Protein also helps stabilize blood sugar levels and prolongs feelings of satiety.

Healthy fats: Olive oil is rich in monounsaturated fatty acids and supports heart health as well as hormonal balance. These healthy fatty acids can also help reduce inflammation.

Hormone support and antioxidants: Pumpkin seeds are rich in zinc and magnesium. Both of these minerals play a critical role in hormone regulation and reducing stress. The antioxidants in the vegetables and seeds protect cells from oxidative damage and support overall health.

TIP

Feel free to add whatever you're in the mood for to make these muffins your own all year long: other vegetables, meat, fish, cheese. . . .

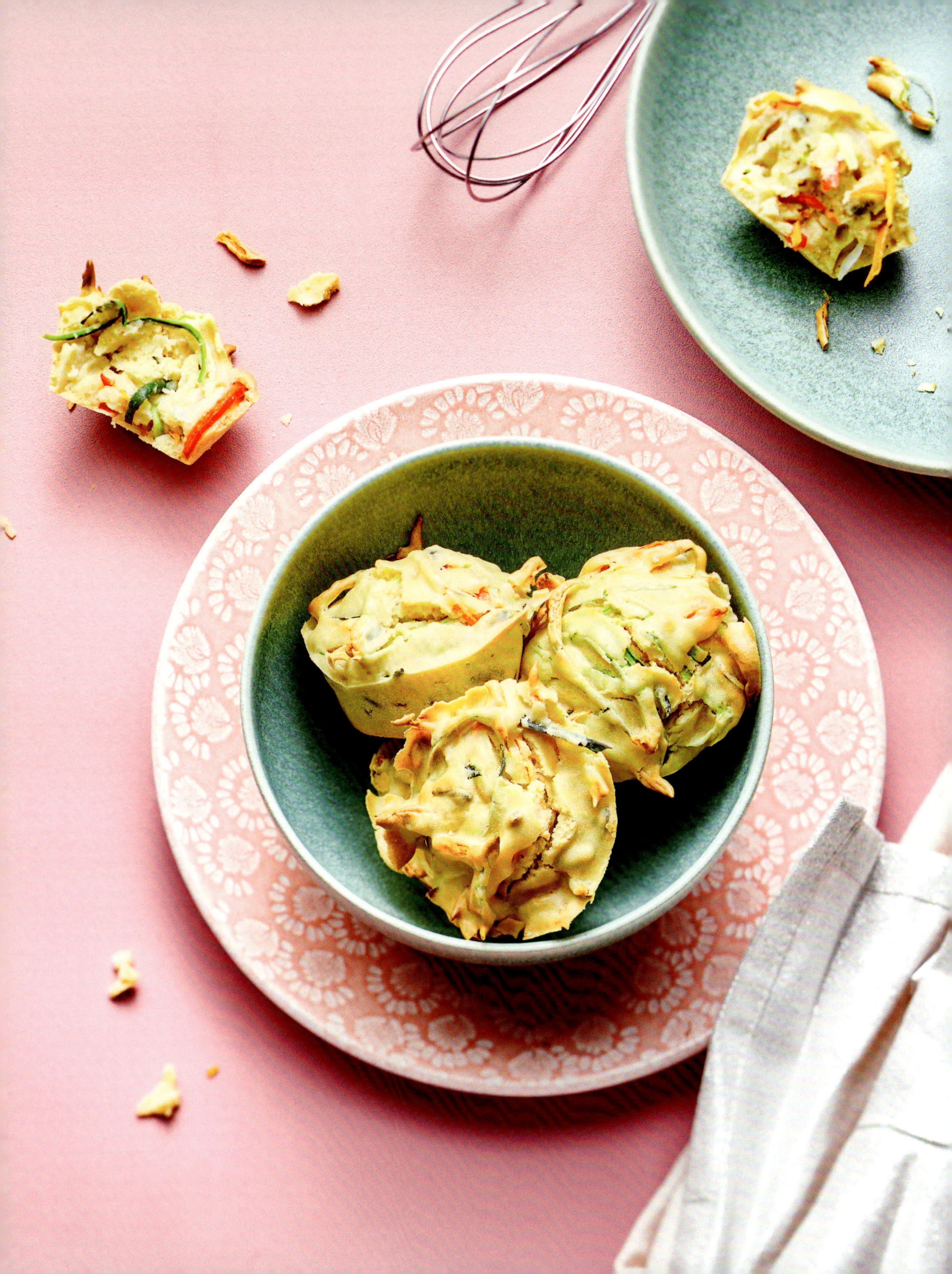

Mushroom-Spinach Omelet

Serves 4
Prep: 5 minutes
Cook: 15 minutes

12 eggs

Salt and pepper

Olive oil (or ghee)

8.8 ounces (250 g) button mushrooms

2 handfuls of fresh spinach

2 stems of fresh chives (or other fresh herbs), chopped

Lettuce

Pumpkin seeds

TIP

Use good-quality eggs (organic if possible) that come from free-range chickens.

RECIPE

Beat the eggs and season with salt and pepper. Heat a drizzle of olive oil in a pan. Next, chop the mushrooms and remove the stalks from the spinach leaves before adding them to the pan. Sauté for around 2 minutes. Pour the beaten eggs over the vegetables and let cook for 2 minutes.

Once the omelet is cooked to your liking, add the chopped herbs and roll the omelet. Serve with a green salad and pumpkin seeds.

HOW IT HELPS YOUR BODY

- **Protein:** Eggs are an excellent source of high-quality protein, which is essential for maintaining muscle mass and supporting cellular regeneration.
- **Vitamins and minerals:** Spinach is rich in vitamins A, C, and K as well as minerals like iron and calcium. These nutrients support bone health and immune function.
- **Antioxidants:** Mushrooms contain antioxidants that combat oxidative stress and reduce inflammation.
- **Fiber:** Although vegetables are used in small quantities in this recipe, they still provide fiber to promote healthy digestion and bowel function.
- **Healthy fatty acids:** The olive oil or ghee in this recipe contains monounsaturated fatty acids that are beneficial for cardiovascular health and hormonal support during menopause.

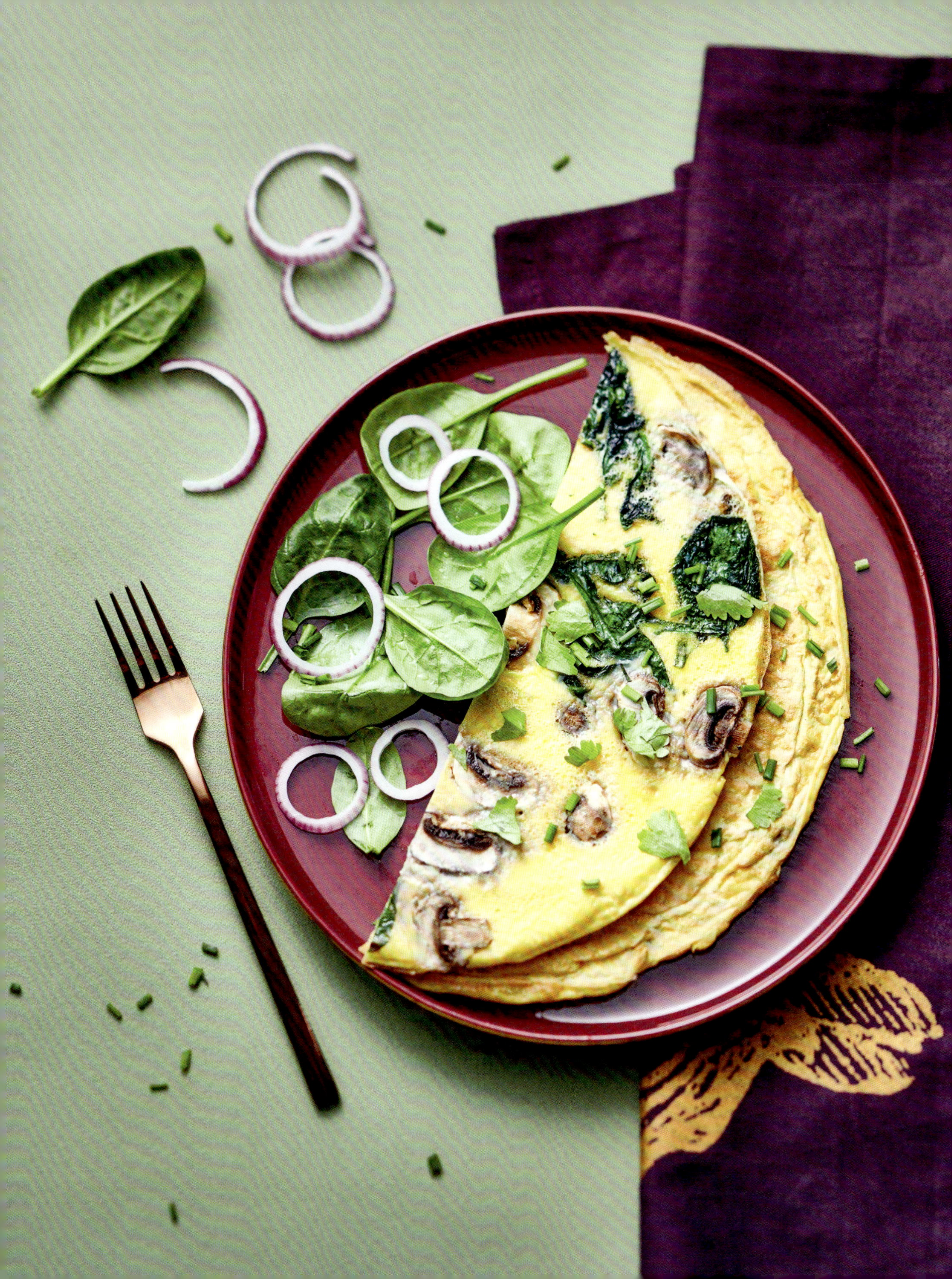

Savory Pancakes with Tuna and Feta

Serves 4
Prep: 10 minutes
Cook: 25 minutes

5.3 ounces (150 g) brown rice flour

1 teaspoon gluten-free baking powder

1 teaspoon sea salt

Pepper, to taste

2 eggs

6.75 fluid ounces (200 ml) plant-based milk

2 tablespoons olive oil (or 1 teaspoon ghee)

5.3 ounces (150 g) canned tuna

3.5 ounces (100 g) feta, crumbled

Fresh parsley, chopped (optional)

TIP

For a balanced meal, serve these pancakes with a green salad or some vegetables on the side.

RECIPE

Mix together the flour, baking powder, salt, and pepper.

Beat the eggs and add the milk and oil. Stir well. Pour the mixture into the flour and stir until fully combined. Drain the tuna and crumble it into the mixture. Add the crumbled feta and chopped parsley. Gently stir to combine.

Heat a pan over medium heat. Add a drizzle of olive oil or ghee. Pour 1 small ladleful of batter into the pan. Cook the pancakes for 2 to 3 minutes on each side until they are golden brown and cooked on the inside.

HOW IT HELPS YOUR BODY

Protein: Tuna and eggs are rich in high-quality protein. This is essential for maintaining muscle mass and supporting tissue regeneration.

Calcium: Feta adds flavor to this recipe and is also a source of calcium. This mineral is crucial for bone health, especially during menopause when the risk of bone loss increases.

Vitamin D: Eggs are a natural source of vitamin D, which helps with calcium absorption and supports bone health. Getting enough vitamin D in your diet is particularly important for preventing osteoporosis and maintaining good bone density.

Minerals: Tuna and feta contain a variety of minerals like magnesium and potassium. These minerals are important for nerve and muscle function as well as electrolyte balance and blood pressure regulation.

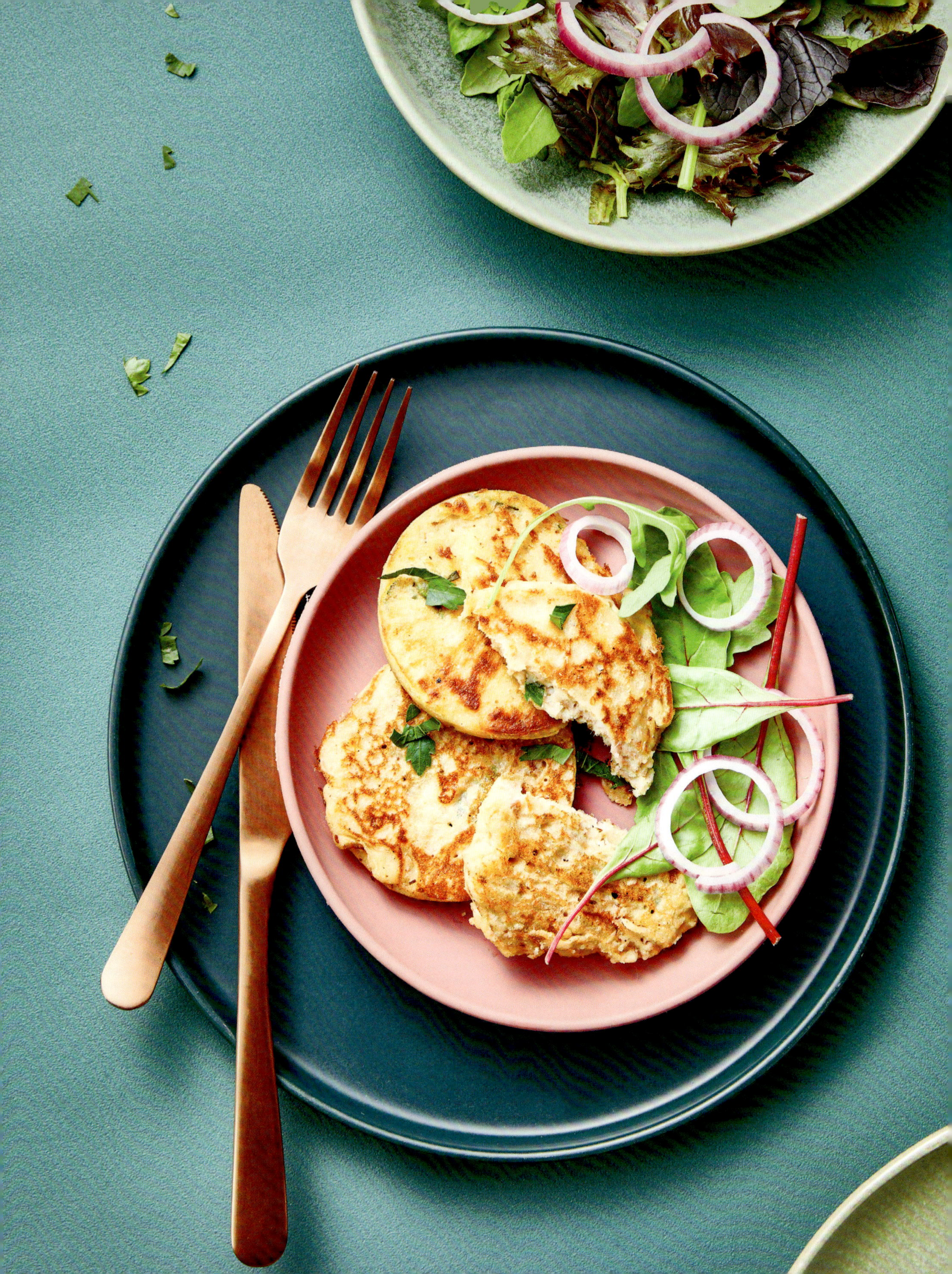

The importance of protein

Proteins are macromolecules made up of amino acids. They can be found in every one of the body's cells and play a crucial role in many of its basic functions. Like the bricks of a house, proteins maintain the structure of the skin, tendons, muscles, hormones, and bones. Without enough protein, everything just falls apart! During menopause, eating the right amount of protein is especially important. This amount will vary depending on factors like a woman's age, weight, level of physical activity, etc., but a general recommendation is 1 to 2 grams of protein for every kilogram of body weight per day (a kilogram is equal to 2.2 pounds).

Protein is important for a number of reasons:

- It helps muscles contract
- It promotes healthy immune function
- It ensures that water and energy are distributed throughout the body
- It preserves muscle mass
- It supports bone health
- It regulates food metabolism
- It contributes to a balanced diet
- It promotes feelings of satiety

How can I get enough protein?

Each of the quantities listed below contains 20 grams of protein.

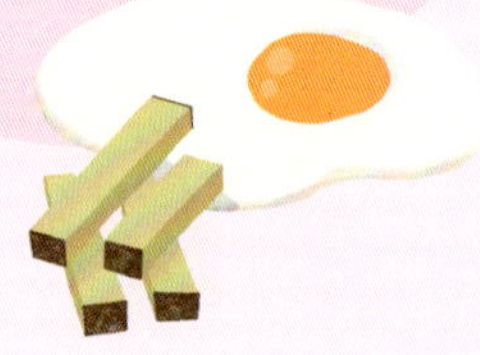

Animal products

2.8 ounces (80 g) tuna
2.8 ounces (80 g) turkey breast
3 ounces (85 g) chicken breast
5 ounces (145 g) whitefish
3.7 ounces (105 g) wild salmon
4.4 ounces (125 g) ham
3.7 ounces (105 g) red meat
3 whole eggs
3.2 ounces (90 g) sardines

Dairy products

4.2 ounces (120 g) feta
2.6 ounces (75 g) Comté
8.8 ounces (250 g) fromage blanc made from sheep or goat's milk
6.3 ounces (180 g) skyr yogurt made from sheep or goat's milk
2.5 ounces (70 g) pecorino
2 ounces (55 g) Parmesan

Grains and legumes

8.8 ounces (250 g) cooked red beans
≈ 4.4 ounces (125 g) dry
8.1 ounces (230 g) cooked lentils
≈ 3.25 ounces (92 g) dry
11 ounces (310 g) cooked chickpeas
≈ 5.5 ounces (155 g) dry
8.8 ounces (250 g) uncooked brown rice
4.6 ounces (130 g) uncooked quinoa
5.3 ounces (150 g) uncooked buckwheat

Other

1 ounce (30 g) spirulina

Seeds and nuts

3.2 ounces (90 g) almonds
3.5 ounces (100 g) pistachios, pumpkin seeds, or chia seeds
2.3 ounces (65 g) hemp seeds
4.6 ounces (130 g) walnuts
3.9 ounces (110 g) cashews
5 ounces (143 g) hazelnuts

Plant-based foods

2.6 ounces (75 g) seitan
23 ounces (650 g) mushrooms
6 ounces (170 g) firm tofu
7 ounces (200 g) silken tofu
3.5 ounces (100 g) tempeh

The idea, of course, is to include lots of different proteins on your plate. The key to nutritional success during menopause lies in a varied diet with as little processed food as possible.

Savory Granola

Makes 1 jar
Prep: 10 minutes
Cook: 30 minutes
Storage: 3 weeks at room temperature

3.5 ounces (100 g) gluten-free oats
2 ounces (60 g) walnuts
2 ounces (60 g) cashews
2 ounces (60 g) pumpkin seeds
1 ounce (30 g) sesame seeds
1 tablespoon fennel seeds
½ teaspoon chili powder
Salt and pepper
1 egg white
4 tablespoons olive oil

RECIPE

Preheat the oven to 350°F (180°C) and line a baking sheet with parchment paper.

Combine the oats, nuts, seeds, and chili powder. Season with salt and pepper. Add the egg white and oil and stir together.

Pour the mixture onto the baking sheet, forming an even layer. Bake for 20 to 30 minutes, stirring 2 or 3 times during baking. Remove from the oven as soon as the granola starts to turn golden brown and let cool on the baking sheet before transferring to an airtight container.

HOW IT HELPS YOUR BODY

- **Proteins and healthy fatty acids:** Seeds and nuts are rich in protein and essential fatty acids. These nutrients help maintain muscle mass, support metabolism, and regulate hormone levels. Essential fatty acids also promote cardiovascular health.
- **Fiber:** Oats and pumpkin seeds contain fiber that is critical for healthy digestion, maintaining stable blood sugar, and weight management.
- **Minerals and antioxidants:** Sesame and fennel seeds provide minerals like calcium and magnesium as well as antioxidants. These nutrients support bone health and help reduce inflammation, which makes it easier to manage certain menopause symptoms.
- **Anti-inflammatory properties:** Fennel seeds are anti-inflammatory and can help reduce joint pain and inflammation.
- **Hormone balance:** Nuts, seeds, and oats are rich in nutrients that support hormonal balance. The healthy fats and minerals in this recipe can help alleviate hormonal symptoms and support overall well-being.

TIP

You can eat this granola as a snack or sprinkle it over salads, soups, or your main dish.

Spinach Salad with Pumpkin Seeds and Tofu

Serves 4
Prep: 15 minutes
Marinate: 15 minutes
Cook: 15 minutes

14 ounces (400 g) firm tofu
1 garlic clove
3 tablespoons tamari
1 tablespoon sesame oil
8.8 ounces (250 g) spinach leaves
6 tablespoons pumpkin seeds
1 avocado, sliced
1 small carrot, grated
1 tablespoon lemon juice
1 tablespoon apple cider vinegar
1 tablespoon maple syrup (or honey)
Salt and pepper

RECIPE

Drain and press the tofu to eliminate excess water. Dice into ½-inch to ¾-inch (1- to 2-cm) cubes. Peel and mince the garlic then combine it with the tamari and sesame oil. Add the tofu cubes and marinate for at least 15 minutes.

Heat a pan over medium heat to cook the marinated tofu until golden and crispy (5 to 7 minutes on each side).

Combine the spinach leaves, pumpkin seeds, sliced avocado, and grated carrot. Whisk together the lemon juice, vinegar, maple syrup, salt, and pepper in a small bowl. Add the tofu cubes, pour the vinaigrette over the salad, and gently toss.

HOW IT HELPS YOUR BODY

- **Protein and amino acids:** Tofu is an excellent source of plant protein. It plays an important role in preserving muscle mass and tissue health. During menopause, eating protein is crucial for supporting your metabolism and energy level.
- **Healthy fats:** Pumpkin seeds are rich in essential fatty acids like omega-3s and omega-6s. These healthy fats promote good cardiovascular health and can help relieve menopause symptoms like hot flashes and hormone imbalance.
- **Vitamins and minerals:** Spinach leaves are an excellent source of vitamins A, C, and K as well as minerals like iron and calcium. These nutrients support bone health, immune function, and hormonal regulation. Avocados contain healthy fats and vitamins, too, which gives this salad an extra nutrient boost!
- **Antioxidants:** Garlic, lemon, and apple cider vinegar provide antioxidants that help fight oxidative stress and reduce inflammation. Antioxidants are important for maintaining cellular health and managing the effects of aging.

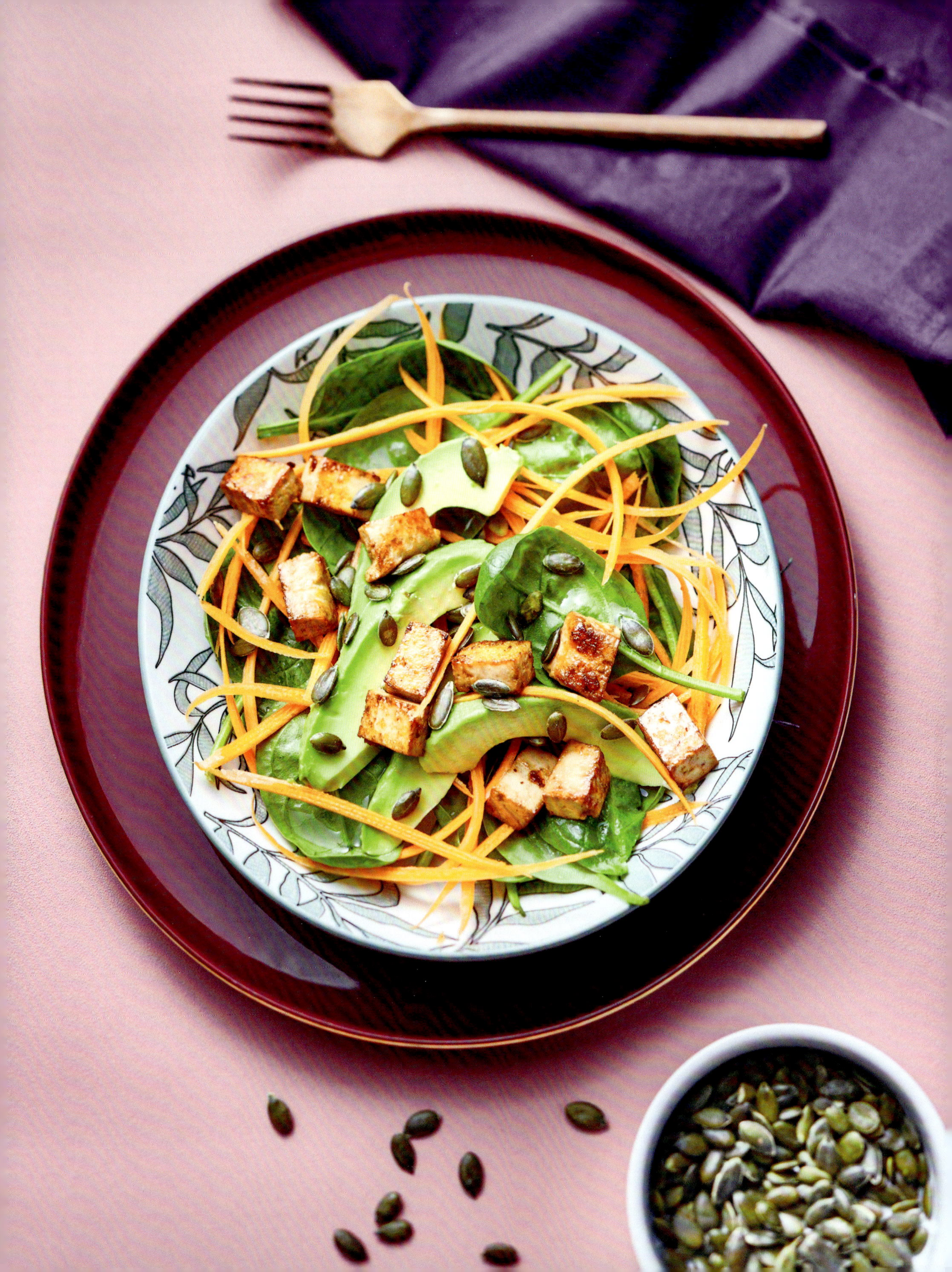

Lentil Salad with Vegetables and Goat Cheese

Serves 4

Lentil soaking: 8 hours (24 hours for sprouted lentils)

Prep: 15 minutes

Cook: 20 minutes

10.5 ounces (300 g) green lentils

14 ounces (400 g) seasonal vegetables (cherry tomatoes, cucumbers, bell peppers, red onions, etc.)

3 tablespoons canola oil

2 tablespoons apple cider vinegar

2 teaspoons Dijon mustard

Salt and black pepper

5.3 ounces (150 g) fresh goat cheese made with raw (unpasteurized) goat's milk

Fresh herbs (parsley, cilantro, basil)

7 ounces (200 g) lettuce or blend of baby lettuces

TIP

If you want to add protein, serve this salad with one or two slices of sourdough bread spread with mackerel rillettes (see recipe page 132).

RECIPE

Soak the lentils the day before, or the morning of, a day you plan to serve this dish for dinner. Soaking makes them tender and easier to digest. It also destroys antinutrients and enhances the lentils' nutritional potential. You can take this even further and let the lentils sprout. This increases the lentils' vitamin and mineral content and makes these nutrients easier to absorb.

The day of, rinse the lentils in cold water and transfer them to a pot with 3 cups (750 ml) of water. Bring to a boil, then lower the heat and let cook for 15 to 20 minutes. Drain and let cool.

While the lentils are cooking, cut the cherry tomatoes in half, dice the cucumbers and peppers, peel and mince the onions, etc.

Combine the oil, vinegar, and mustard, then season this mixture with salt and pepper.

Combine the lentils and vegetables in a large bowl. Add crumbled goat cheese and chopped herbs. Pour over the vinaigrette and gently toss. Divide the baby lettuce or lettuce leaves between the plates and add the lentil salad on top before serving.

HOW IT HELPS YOUR BODY

Protein and fiber: Lentils are an excellent source of plant protein and fiber. They help maintain muscle mass and promote healthy digestion. Fiber helps regulate bowel function and maintain a healthy weight.

Vitamins and minerals: Fresh vegetables like cherry tomatoes, cucumbers, and peppers are rich in vitamins A, C, and K as well as potassium and magnesium. These nutrients support the immune system, bone health, and blood pressure regulation. Goat cheese provides calcium, which is important for bone health.

Antioxidants: Brightly colored vegetables are full of antioxidants that help combat oxidative stress and reduce inflammation. These antioxidants are especially beneficial during menopause to counter the effects of cell aging and support overall health.

Healthy fats: The canola oil used in the vinaigrette is rich in omega-3 fatty acids that are beneficial for cardiovascular health. Omega-3s also help reduce inflammation and support hormonal balance.

Probiotics and digestion: Apple cider vinegar aids digestion and maintains healthy gut flora. Healthy digestion is essential for nutrient absorption and general well-being.

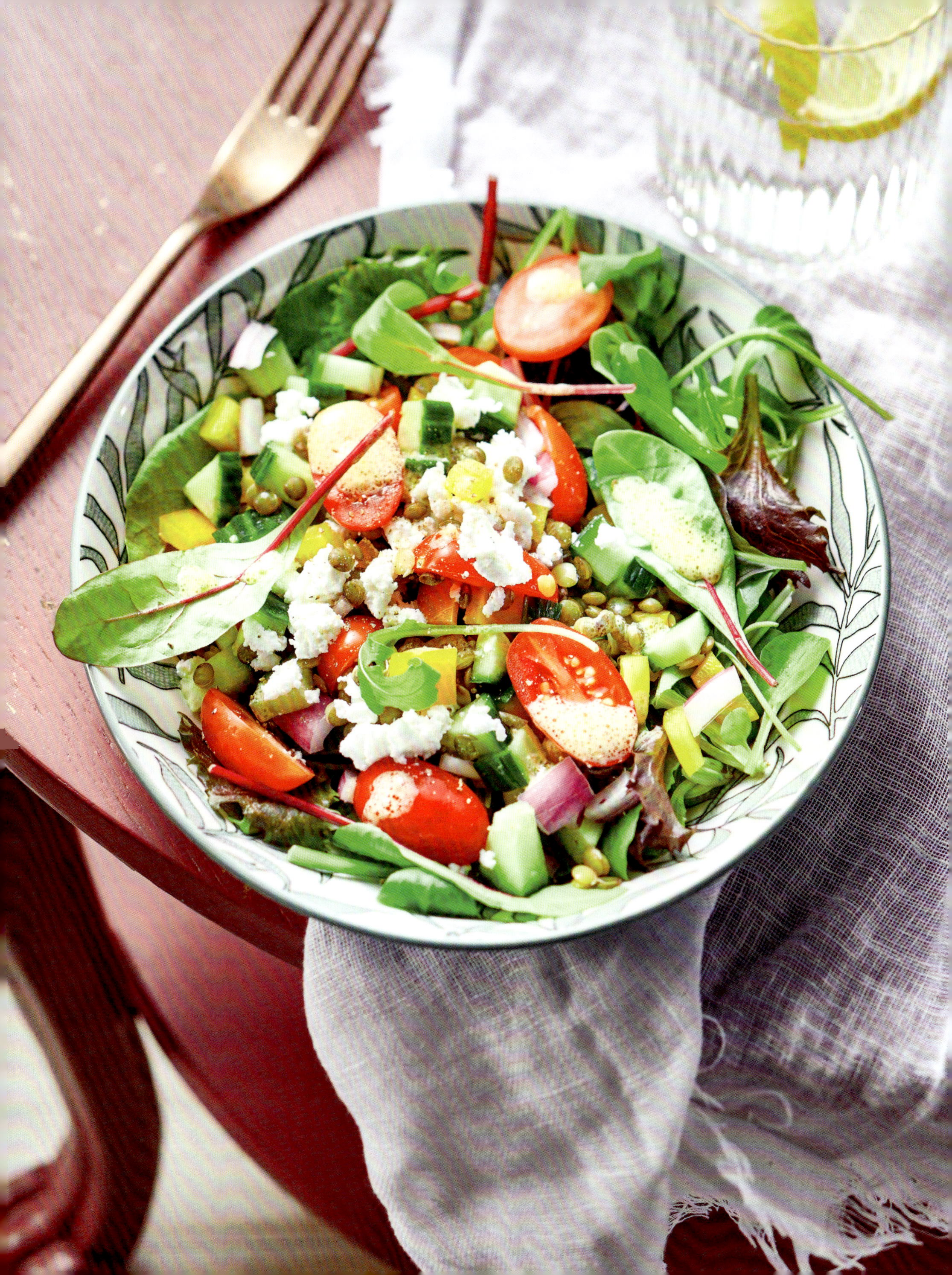

Stuffed Eggplant with Silken Tofu

Serves 4
Prep: 20 minutes
Cook: 50 minutes

2 eggplants

2 tablespoons olive oil

Salt and pepper

7 ounces (200 g) silken tofu

2 garlic cloves

3.5 ounces (100 g) Parmesan, grated or shaved, divided

2 tablespoons tamari

3 pinches dried oregano

Fresh cilantro

Green salad

RECIPE

Preheat the oven to 350°F (180°C).

Cut the eggplants in half lengthwise. Score the flesh of each piece of eggplant with a knife to make a diamond crosshatch pattern. Drizzle the eggplant halves with oil, season with salt and pepper, and arrange on a baking tray. Bake for 30 to 35 minutes.

Crush the tofu with a fork until you have a smooth consistency. Peel and chop the garlic and add that to the tofu along with half of the Parmesan, the tamari, oregano, salt, and pepper and stir together.

Once the eggplant is cooked, use a spoon to gently hollow out each eggplant half. Add the cooked eggplant flesh to the tofu and stir until combined. Now fill each eggplant half with this mixture.

Sprinkle the rest of the Parmesan over the eggplant halves and put them back in the oven for 10 to 15 minutes. Serve with chopped cilantro and salad.

HOW IT HELPS YOUR BODY

Plant proteins: Silken tofu provides high-quality plant protein that is essential for preserving muscle mass and regenerating tissue in the body.

Calcium and vitamin D: Parmesan is a good source of calcium, which is necessary for bone health. It is particularly important to make sure you're getting enough calcium during menopause to prevent bone density loss.

Antioxidants and anti-inflammatories: Garlic and oregano contain antioxidant and anti-inflammatory compounds. These compounds help reduce oxidative stress and inflammation, strengthen the immune system, and support overall well-being.

Fiber: Eggplant is high in fiber, which promotes healthy digestion and regular bowel movements. Fiber also helps with weight management and feeling full after eating.

Healthy fats: Olive oil contains monounsaturated fatty acids that are beneficial for cardiovascular health. These fatty acids can help balance cholesterol levels and support hormonal health.

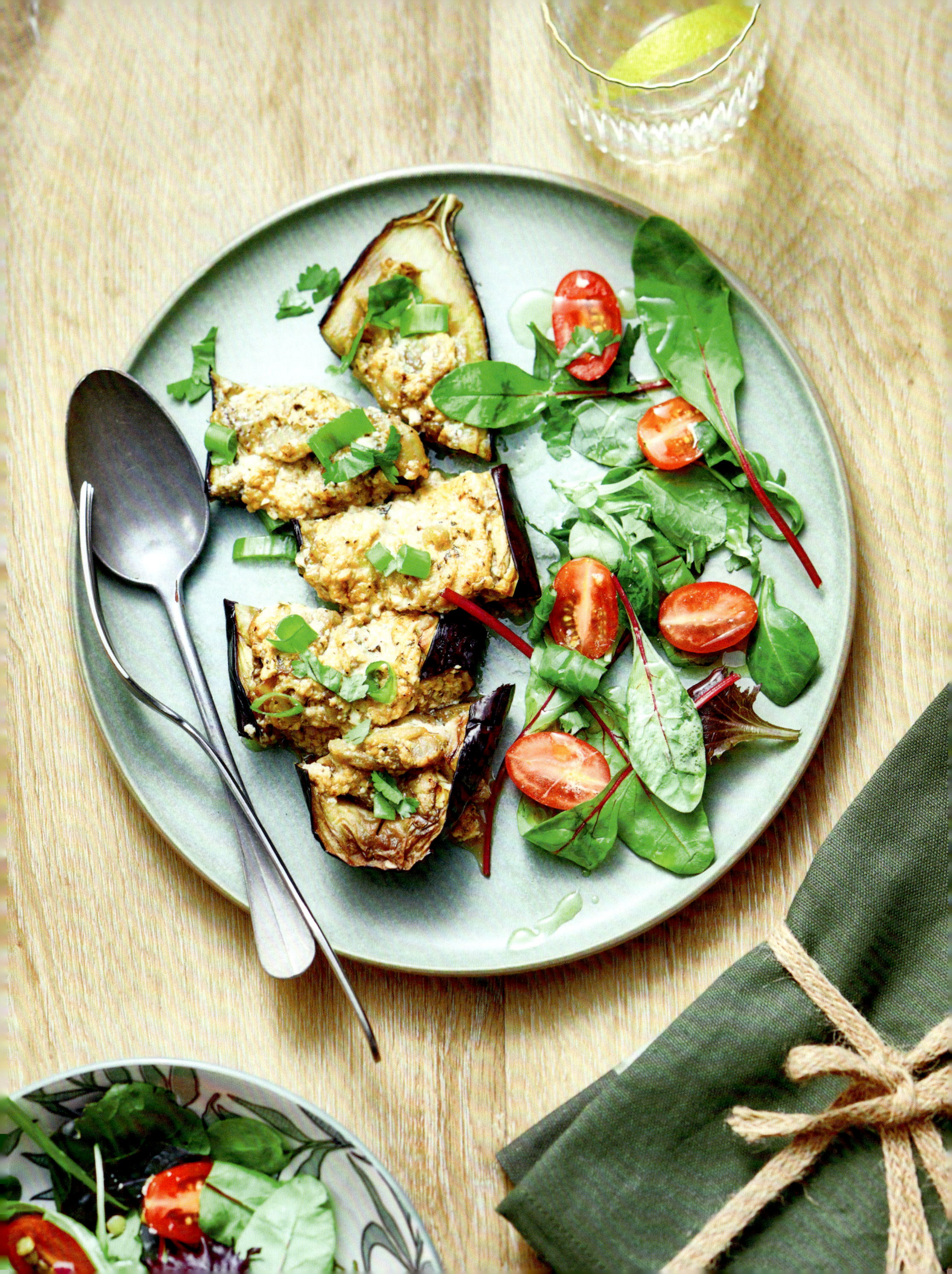

Marinated Tofu and Vegetable Kebabs

Serves 4
Prep: 15 minutes
Marinate: 30 minutes
Cook: 25 minutes

For the marinade:

4 tablespoons tamari

2 tablespoons olive oil

2 garlic cloves, minced

1 teaspoon fresh ginger, grated (optional)

Salt and pepper

14 ounces (400 g) firm tofu

2 zucchini

2 bell peppers (red, yellow, or green)

1 red onion

TIP

You can serve these kebabs with whole-grain rice, quinoa, or a green salad.

RECIPE

Combine the marinade ingredients.

Cut the tofu into cubes and place in a shallow dish. Pour over the marinade and let sit for at least 30 minutes in the refrigerator.

Preheat the oven to 350°F (180°C).

Slice the zucchini into rounds, chop the peppers, and peel and quarter the onion. Now assemble the kebabs. Thread the tofu cubes onto the skewers, alternating with zucchini rounds, chunks of pepper, and pieces of onion. Place kebabs on a baking sheet lined with parchment paper and bake for 20 to 25 minutes, turning over halfway through cooking, until the vegetables are tender and the tofu is golden brown.

HOW IT HELPS YOUR BODY

- **Plant protein:** Tofu is an excellent source of plant protein. It also contains isoflavones, which are phytoestrogens that can help alleviate menopause symptoms.
- **Vitamins and minerals:** Zucchini, peppers, and onions are rich in vitamins and essential minerals. Zucchini contains potassium as well as vitamins A and C. Peppers are an excellent source of vitamin C, which is important for the immune system and skin health. Onions provide antioxidants and anti-inflammatory compounds that support overall health and reduce inflammation symptoms.
- **Antioxidants:** Garlic and ginger both have antioxidant and anti-inflammatory properties. They help combat oxidative stress and inflammation to improve energy levels and relieve menopause symptoms.
- **Healthy fats:** The olive oil in the marinade is a source of monounsaturated fatty acids, which promote cardiovascular health and regulate cholesterol levels in the blood.
- **Fiber:** The vegetables in this recipe are full of fiber, which contributes to healthy digestion and helps the body maintain stable blood sugar levels. Fiber is also important in weight management and supporting metabolic balance. This can be useful for managing hormonal fluctuations and overall well-being.

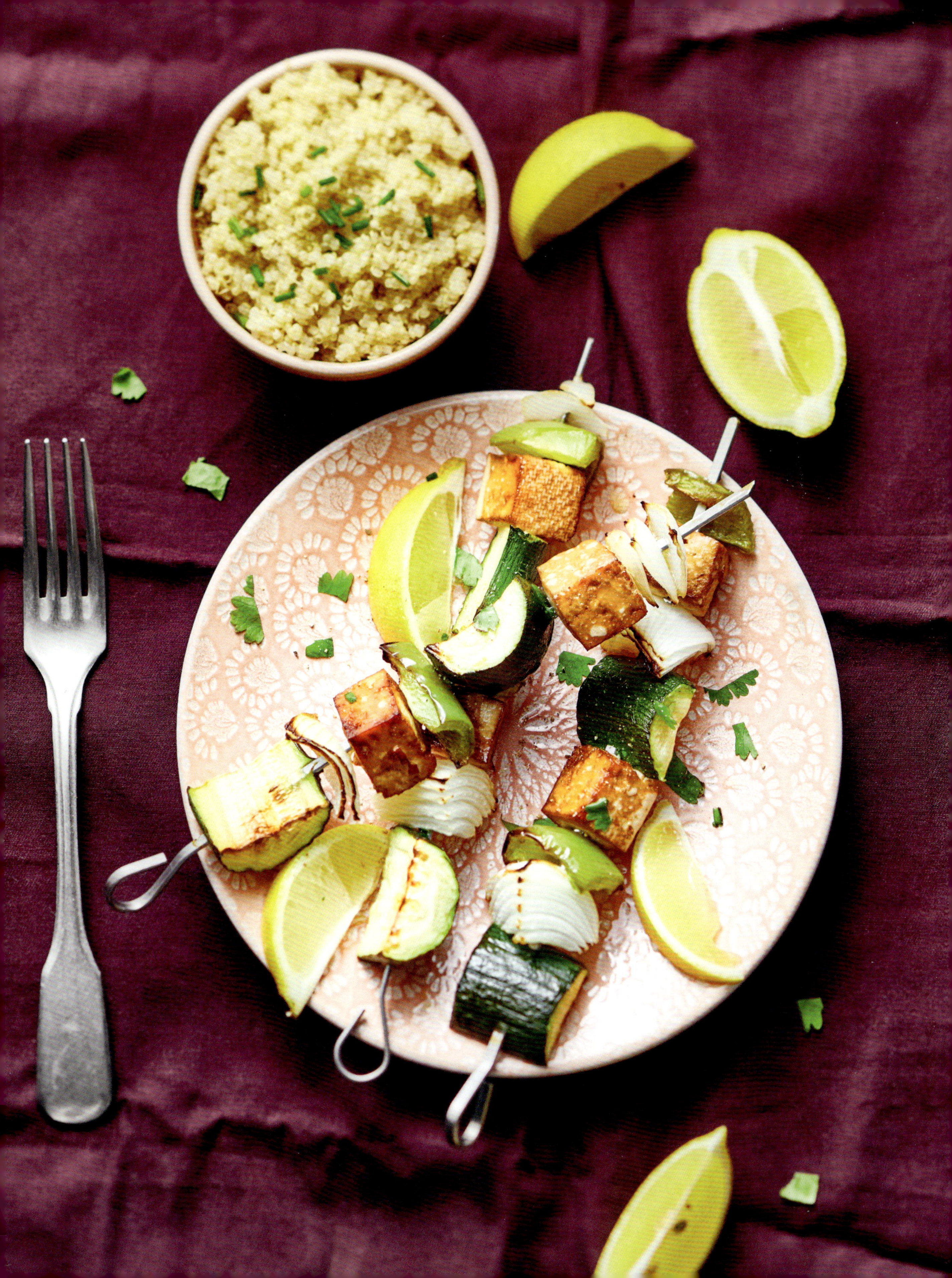

Soy

There has been somewhat of a divergence of opinion on soy in the past several years. Unfortunately, this makes it easy to forget soy's nutritional benefits—especially before, during, and after menopause. Studies on the subject are often contradictory. Part of the reason for this is that these studies often do not take into account certain essential parameters that influence soy's nutritional value: product traceability, the quantity consumed per day, and preparation methods (raw, cooked, fermented, or sprouted).

Soy possesses undeniable nutritional benefits, but it also contains compounds that can be problematic for your health if eaten in excess, if the soy is low quality, or if the soy is prepared in a way that makes it difficult to digest (raw, unfermented, or not sprouted, for instance).

What's the best way to eat soy?

In small quantities:

Sprouts

Soybean sprouts
Mung bean sprouts

Fermented

Natto
Miso
Lacto-fermented tofu
Tempeh
Tamari

Soy milk

Use in cooking to replace cow's milk

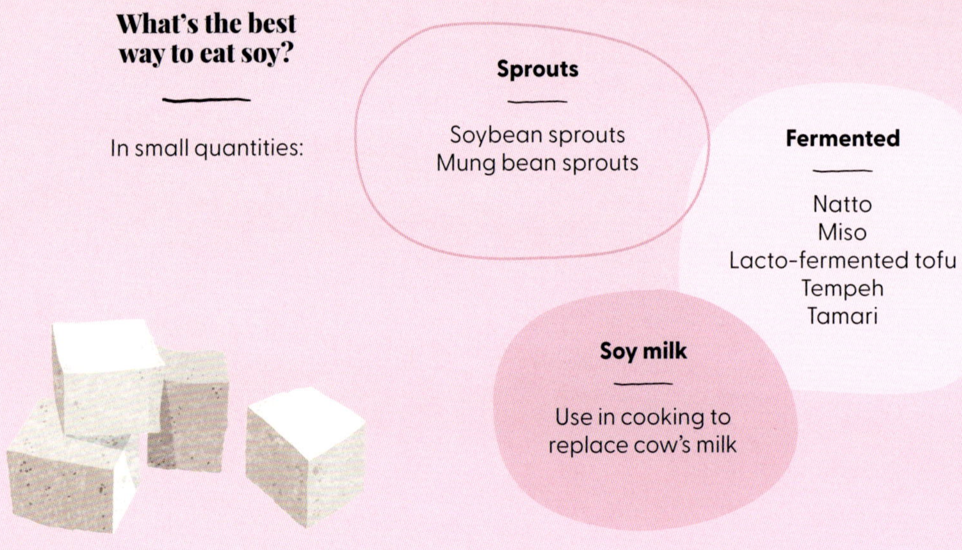

Phytoestrogens

Phytoestrogens are natural compounds found in certain plant foods like soy, oats, chickpeas, clover, flaxseed, green beans, parsley, garlic, sesame, corn, cucumber, anisette, olives, beets, papaya, sunflower seeds, wheat germ, lentils, alfalfa, olive oil, and more.

They mimic what estrogen does in the body without having the same significant effects.

Think of phytoestrogens as a crutch to lean on during the menopause transition and all of its hormonal fluctuations. Eating more phytoestrogens ahead of and during menopause limits bone demineralization and reduces hot flashes.

How should I cook tofu?

If you're not familiar with this ingredient already, here are a few tips:

Drain and press the tofu in a paper towel to remove excess water. This will allow the tofu to absorb more flavor.

Marinate it: Tofu has a neutral flavor and can be used in a variety of ways.

A few ideas for marinades

Asian: tamari, grated fresh ginger, minced garlic, sesame oil

Curry: curry paste (red, yellow, or green), coconut milk, tamari, grated fresh ginger

Mediterranean: olive oil, lemon juice, dried oregano, chopped fresh basil, minced garlic

Orange-ginger: fresh orange juice, grated fresh ginger, tamari, sesame oil

Tomato-basil: tomato purée, chopped fresh basil, minced garlic, balsamic vinegar

Cooking methods

Stir-fry: Sauté the tofu in a pan with a little bit of oil until it is golden and crispy.

Grilled: Use a grill or pan to get it crispy on the outside and still tender on the inside.

Oven-roasted: Slice or cut into cubes and bake in the oven until golden and crispy. Turn the tofu over halfway through baking to make sure it is cooked evenly.

Serving ideas

Stir-fry: Add tofu to your vegetable stir-fries for some plant-based protein.

Salad: Add grilled or marinated tofu to your salads for more texture and flavor.

Curry: Tofu pairs well with spicy curry sauces. Add it to your curry dishes for a vegetarian alternative.

Grain bowls: Use tofu as a main ingredient in grain bowls with vegetables and other protein for a balanced meal.

Chickpea Curry with Cashews

Serves 4
Prep: 5 minutes
Cook: 15 minutes

1 onion

1 garlic clove

Olive oil

8.8 ounces (250 g) cooked chickpeas (4.4 ounces [125 g] dry)

6.75 fluid ounces (200 ml) tomato purée

1 teaspoon tomato paste

6.75 fluid ounces (200 ml) coconut milk

3 teaspoons curry powder

Salt and pepper

2 heaping tablespoon cashew butter

Rice or quinoa, prepared for serving

Raw cashews

Fresh cilantro

Green salad

RECIPE

Peel the onion and garlic. Thinly slice the onion, mince the garlic, and sauté both in a pan with a drizzle of olive oil for around 3 minutes. Add the chickpeas, tomato purée, tomato paste, coconut milk, curry powder, salt, pepper, and cashew butter. Stir everything together and let simmer for around 10 minutes.

Serve with rice or quinoa, chopped cashews, chopped cilantro, and salad.

HOW IT HELPS YOUR BODY

- **Plant proteins:** Chickpeas are an excellent source of plant protein, which is essential for maintaining muscle mass and supporting tissue regeneration. Protein also makes weight management easier because it helps you feel full.
- **Calcium and magnesium:** Cashew butter and coconut milk contain calcium and magnesium. Calcium helps maintain bone density and magnesium supports muscle and nerve function.
- **Antioxidants and vitamins:** Garlic and cilantro are rich in antioxidants, which help battle oxidative stress and inflammation. They can also improve overall well-being and support the immune system.
- **Fiber:** Chickpeas provide fiber, which is important for healthy digestion and regular bowel movements. Fiber also contributes to weight management and stable energy levels.
- **Calming effects:** Cashews and coconut milk contain creamy, healthy fats that are beneficial for cardiovascular health and hormonal balance.

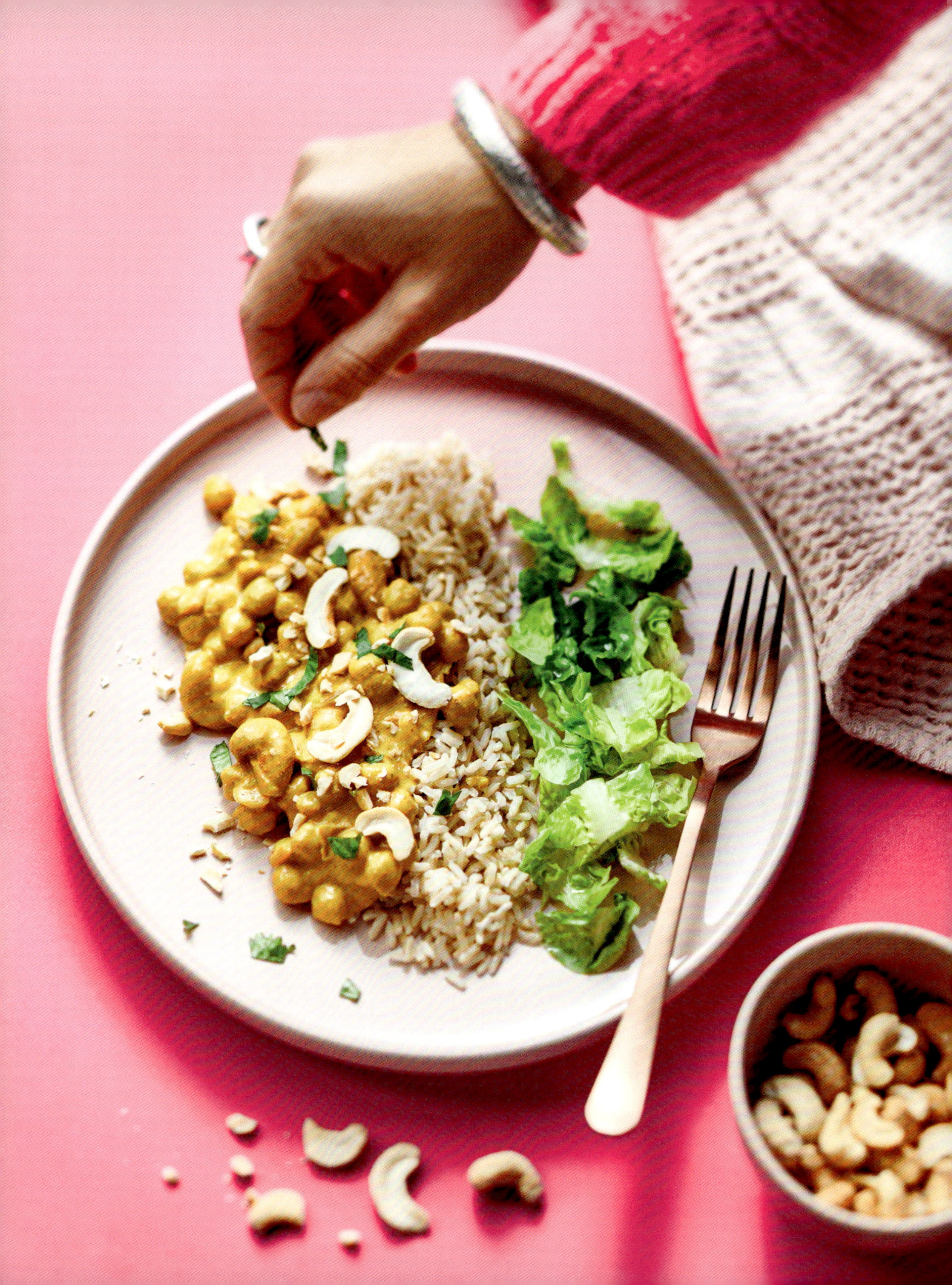

Quinoa with Tempeh and Vegetables

Serves 4
Soak: 2 hours
Prep: 20 minutes
Cook: 20 to 25 minutes

10.5 ounces (300 g) quinoa
2 tablespoons olive oil
1 onion
3 garlic cloves
10.5 ounces (300 g) tempeh
1 carrot
4 tablespoons tamari
2 teaspoons ground turmeric
1 teaspoon ground ginger
Salt and pepper
Fresh parsley

Spring/Summer Version:
2 zucchini
2 red bell peppers

Autumn/Winter Version:
1 parsnip
1 small cauliflower

RECIPE

If you can, soak the quinoa for 2 hours (1 or 2 days if you want it sprouted). Rinse thoroughly and cook in a pot of boiling water (1 part quinoa to 2 parts water) for around 10 minutes until all of the water is absorbed. Cover and leave to rest.

While the quinoa cooks, heat 2 tablespoons of oil over medium heat. Peel and mince the onion and garlic, then sauté together in the pan for a few minutes. Cut the tempeh into cubes and add to the pan. Cook for around 5 minutes until golden. Peel the carrot, slice it into rounds, and dice the other vegetables. Add these to the pan and cook until tender (7 to 10 minutes for summer vegetables and 10 to 12 minutes for winter vegetables).

Add the tamari, turmeric, and ginger, followed by the cooked quinoa. Stir well and cook for 2 to 3 minutes. Season with salt and pepper and garnish with chopped parsley or other fresh herbs. Serve hot.

HOW IT HELPS YOUR BODY

- **Complete proteins:** Quinoa and tempeh are sources of complete protein. This means they provide all of the essential amino acids that are needed for preserving muscle mass and the body's metabolism.
- **Digestive support:** Quinoa is rich in fiber, which promotes healthy digestion and helps maintain regular bowel function.
- **Anti-inflammatory properties:** Turmeric and ginger are well-known anti-inflammatories that can help relieve joint pain and inflammation.
- **Vitality and energy:** Seasonal vegetables and olive oil contain vitamins, minerals, and essential antioxidants that help maintain energy and vitality (not to mention healthy fats for the heart!).
- **Hormonal balance:** Tempeh is made from fermented soybeans and contains isoflavones that support hormonal equilibrium and relieve certain menopause symptoms.

MARINADE IDEAS

For a miso flavor, you can marinate the tempeh for a few hours in the refrigerator with 2 tablespoons of miso paste, 3 tablespoons of water, 1 tablespoon of rice vinegar, 1 tablespoon of maple syrup, 1 teaspoon of grated fresh ginger, and 1 teaspoon of sesame oil.

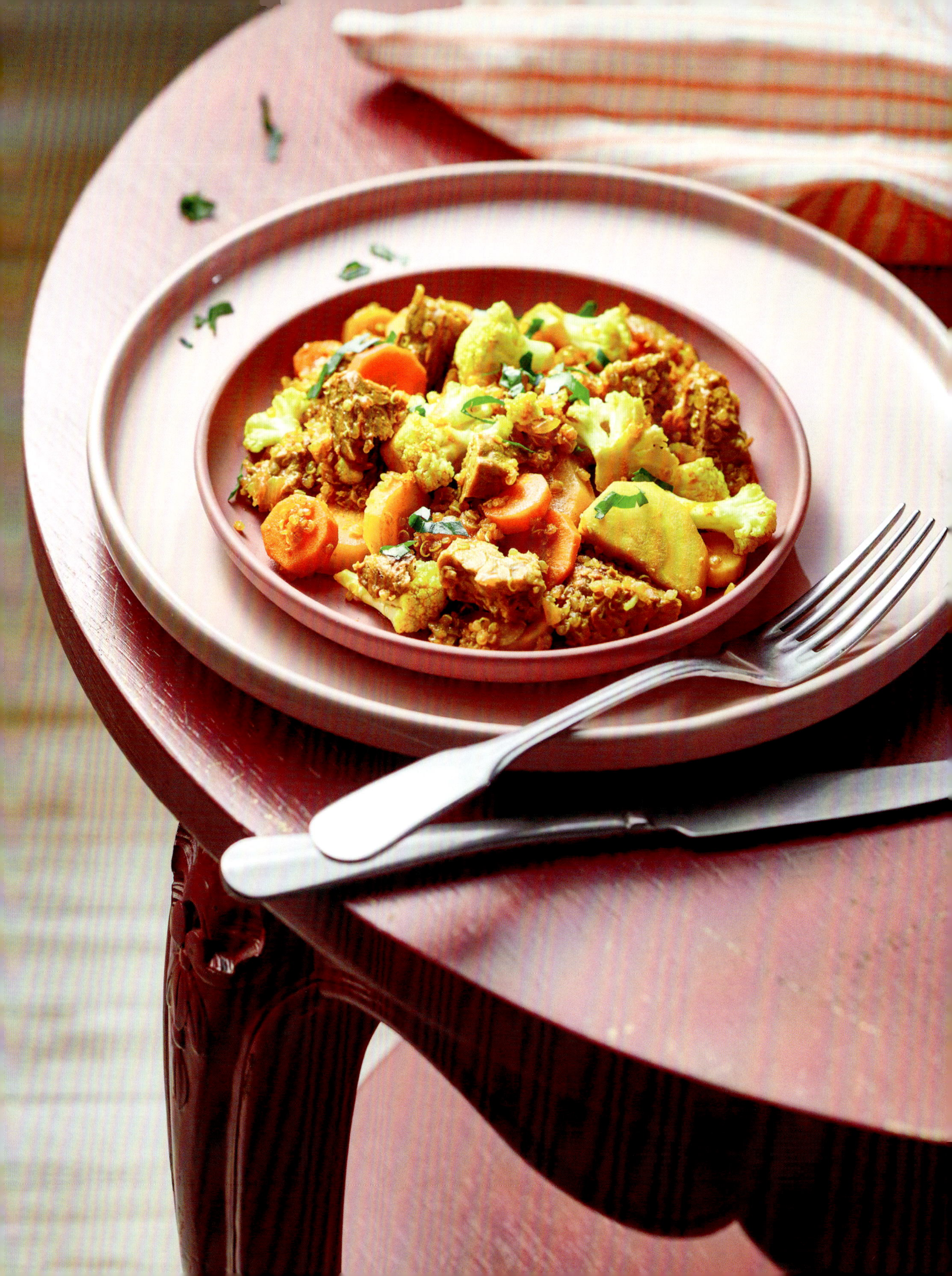

Vegetarian Lentil Pasta

Serves 4
Soak: 10 minutes
Prep: 15 minutes
Cook: 30 minutes

Water or vegetable broth

1.75 ounces (50 g) textured soy protein (+ water or vegetable broth)

2 tablespoons olive oil

1 onion

2 garlic cloves

1 carrot

1 celery stalk

3.5 ounces (100 g) cooked lentils (green or brown)

14 ounces (400 g) crushed tomatoes

1 teaspoon dried oregano

1 teaspoon dried basil

Salt and pepper

10.5 ounces (300 g) semi- or whole-grain spaghetti

1.75 ounces (50 g) Parmesan, grated

RECIPE

In a bowl, pour hot water or vegetable broth over the textured soy protein until it is completely covered. Let sit for 10 minutes, then drain and press to remove any excess liquid.

Heat the oil over medium heat in a large pan or pot. Peel and finely chop the onion and add it to the pan. Cook until the pieces of onion are translucent (around 5 minutes).

Peel and finely chop the garlic and dice the carrot and celery. Add all three to the pan and cook for 5 to 7 minutes until the vegetables are tender. Add the soy protein and cooked lentils. Cook for 2 to 3 minutes. Add the tomatoes, oregano, and basil. Stir everything together and let simmer for 15 minutes over low heat. Season with salt and pepper as needed.

While the sauce is cooking, cook the spaghetti in a large pot of salted boiling water following the instructions on the packet (usually 8 to 10 minutes for semi-whole wheat or whole wheat pasta). Drain the pasta and stir it into the vegetable sauce. Serve hot with Parmesan.

HOW IT HELPS YOUR BODY

- **Complete protein:** Textured soy proteins and lentils offer a plant-based source of complete protein. This helps maintain muscle mass and regulate metabolism.
- **Digestive fiber:** Lentils and semi-whole or whole wheat pasta contain fiber that promotes healthy digestion and regular bowel function.
- **Antioxidants:** Tomatoes are rich in lycopene, an antioxidant that helps protect cells from oxidative damage and supports overall health.
- **Balanced blood sugar:** Semi-whole and whole wheat pasta have a lower glycemic index, which helps stabilize blood sugar and avoid insulin spikes. This is an important part of weight management and hormonal health.
- **Cardiovascular support:** Olive oil and Parmesan contain healthy fats and nutrients that support heart health.

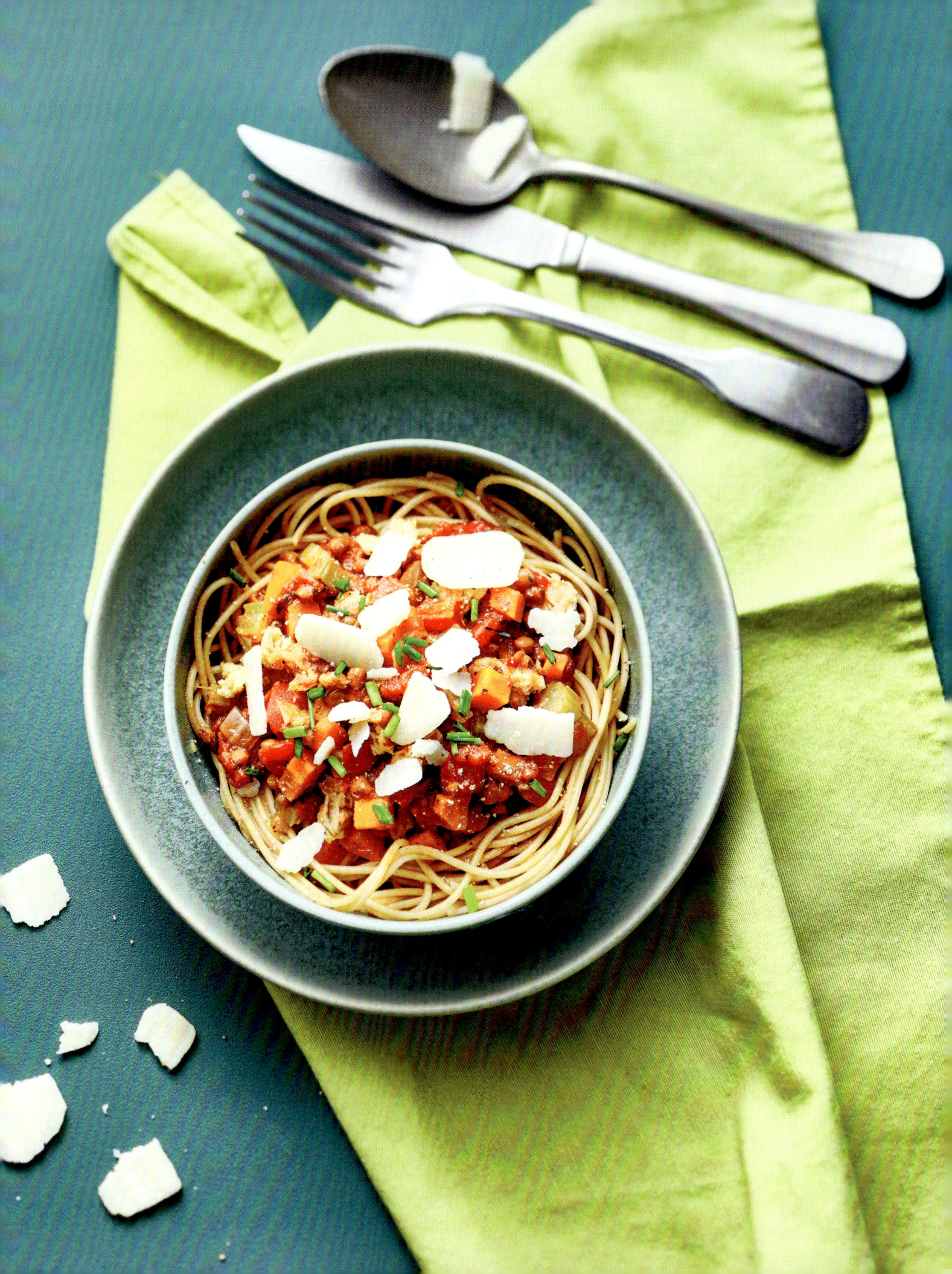

Tofu Vegetable Stir-Fry

Serves 4
Prep: 15 minutes
Cook: 20 minutes

14 ounces (400 g) firm tofu

2 tablespoons tamari

1 tablespoon rice vinegar

1 tablespoon maple syrup (or honey)

1 tablespoon sesame oil

2 garlic cloves

¾-inch (2 cm) piece fresh ginger

7 ounces (200 g) green beans

7 ounces (200 g) sugar snap peas

2 bok choy

1 teaspoon red pepper flakes

Sesame seeds

1 green onion

RECIPE

Drain and press the tofu to remove any excess water. Cut into ¾-inch (2 cm) cubes.

Combine the tamari, vinegar, and maple syrup.

Heat the oil over medium-high heat in a large pan or wok. Sauté the tofu cubes until golden brown and crispy on all sides (5 to 7 minutes). Remove the tofu from the pan.

Add more oil to the pan if necessary. Peel and mince the garlic and grate the ginger. Add both to the pan and sauté for around 1 minute. Trim the green beans and cut into 2-inch (5 cm) pieces. Add to the pan and cook for 5 minutes until they are just about tender. Add the sugar snap peas and cook for another 2 to 3 minutes. Slice the bok choy lengthwise into strips and add to the pan. Cook until tender (2 to 3 minutes).

Return the tofu to the pan of vegetables. Pour in the sauce. Stir well, add the red pepper flakes, and cook for another 2 to 3 minutes to warm everything through and to allow the flavors to intermingle. Sprinkle with sesame seeds and chopped green onion.

HOW IT HELPS YOUR BODY

- **Protein:** Firm tofu is an excellent source of plant protein. This is critical for maintaining muscle mass and regulating hormones.
- **Fiber and antioxidants:** Green vegetables contain fiber and antioxidants that support digestion and cell defense.
- **Balanced blood sugar:** Maple syrup or honey will add a touch of natural sweetness, but we've only included a small amount in this recipe to avoid upsetting blood glucose levels.
- **Anti-inflammatory properties:** Ginger and garlic's anti-inflammatory properties can help reduce symptoms related to inflammation.
- **Healthy fats:** Sesame oil contains healthy fats and nutrients that are important for cardiovascular support and general health.

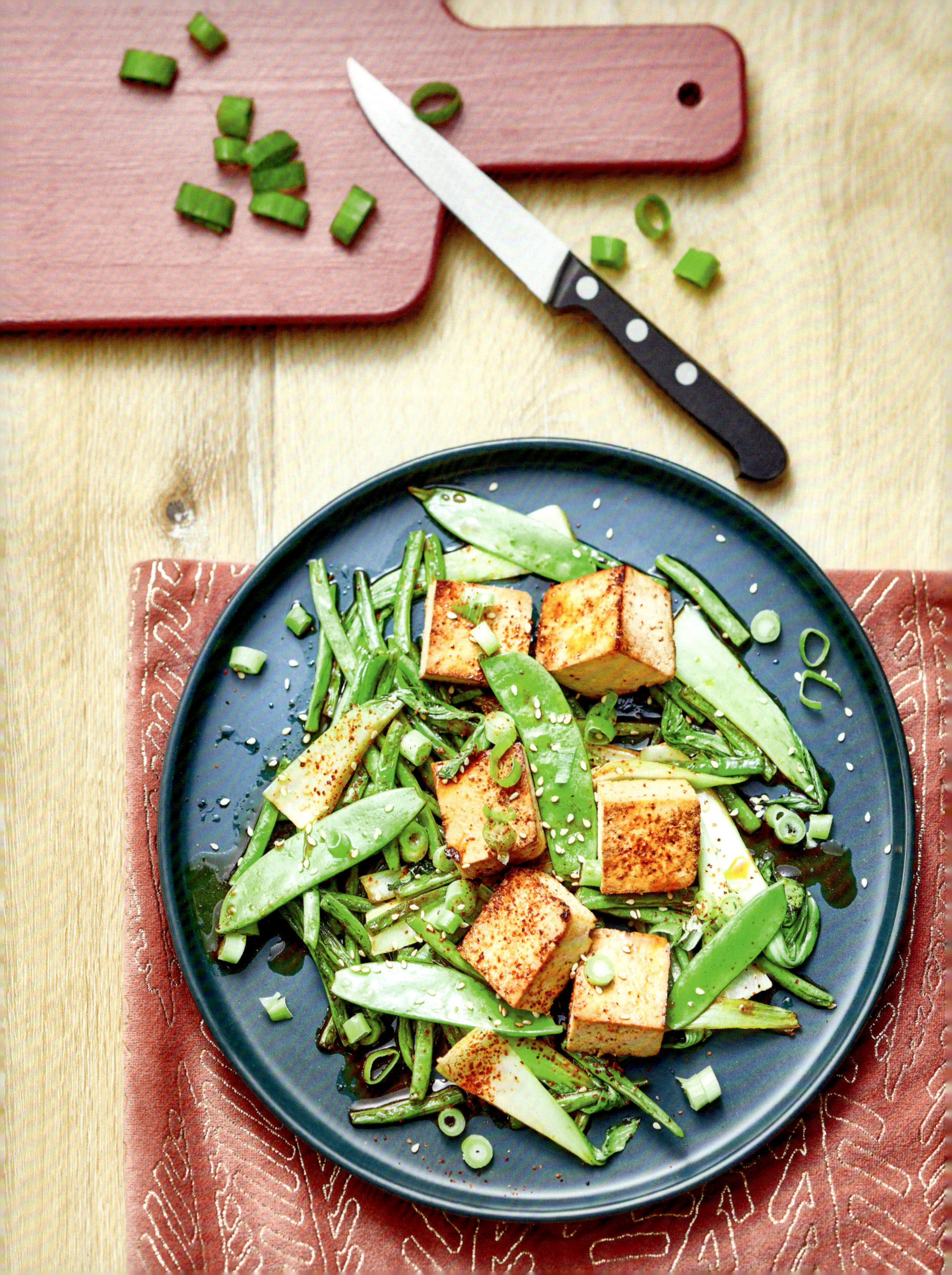

Walnut-Crusted Fish with Roasted Vegetables

Serves 4
Prep: 15 minutes
Cook: 25 minutes

Autumn/Winter Version:

2 carrots

1 parsnip

1 turnip

1 red onion

2 garlic cloves

Spring/Summer Version:

2 zucchini

2 bell peppers (red, yellow, or green)

1 red onion

2 garlic cloves

Olive oil

Fresh herbs (thyme, rosemary, parsley)

Salt and pepper

2 garlic cloves

Juice of 2 lemons

4 whitefish fillets (cod, hake, sea bass . . .)

3.5 ounces (100 g) chopped walnuts

RECIPE

Preheat the oven to 350°F (180°C).

Thinly slice the vegetables or cut into rounds or cubes. Spread them out on a baking sheet. Drizzle with 2 tablespoons of olive oil, sprinkle over the herbs, and season with salt and pepper. Toss to combine and bake for 20 to 25 minutes until tender and starting to brown.

Peel and thinly slice the garlic. Combine with the lemon juice, 2 tablespoons of oil, and chopped herbs. Season with salt and pepper. Generously slather each fish fillet with this mixture. Coat each fillet in chopped nuts and place on a baking sheet lined with parchment paper. Bake alongside the vegetables for 15 to 20 minutes until the fish is cooked and the crust is golden brown.

HOW IT HELPS YOUR BODY

- **Protein:** Whitefish offers an excellent source of lean protein, which is crucial for maintaining muscle mass and managing weight during menopause.
- **Healthy fats:** Nuts contain omega-3 fatty acids. These are beneficial for heart health and help reduce the inflammation that can build up during menopause.
- **Vitamins and minerals:** The roasted vegetables provide vitamins A, C, and K as well as minerals like potassium. These nutrients support bone heath and blood pressure regulation.
- **Antioxidants:** Using fresh herbs and lemon in the marinade provides antioxidants that help fight oxidative stress and promote overall health.
- **Digestive support:** Olive oil, rich in monounsaturated fatty acids, improves digestion and helps maintain gut health.

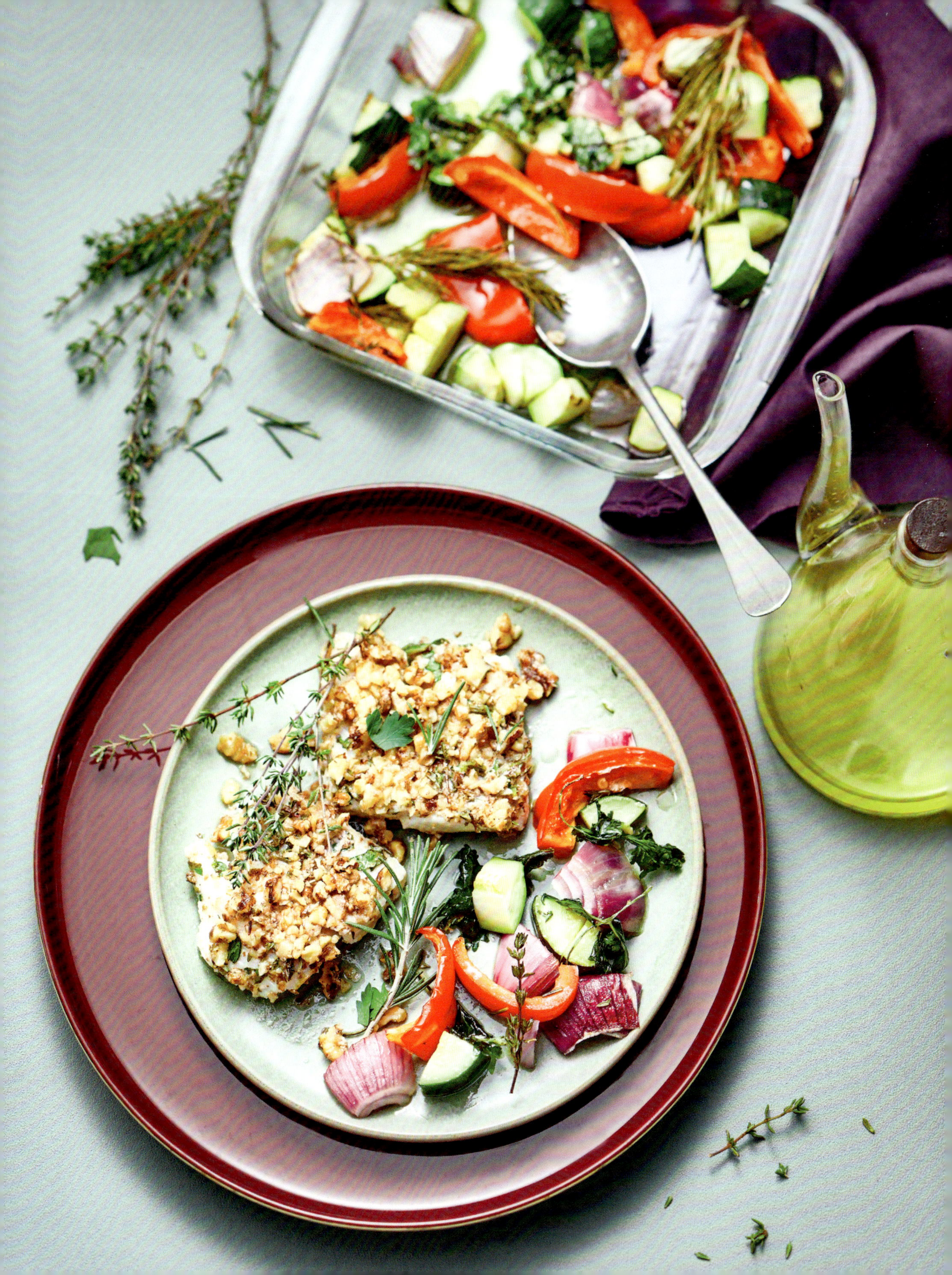

Banana Flaxseed Smoothie

Serves 1
Prep: 5 minutes

8 fluid ounces (250 ml) plant-based milk

1 banana

1 tablespoon ground flaxseed

RECIPE

Combine all ingredients in a blender and blend until smooth. Serve immediately.

HOW IT HELPS YOUR BODY

- **Fiber and digestion:** Ground flaxseed is rich in fiber, which promotes healthy digestion and prevents constipation.
- **Omega-3 fatty acids:** Flaxseed is an excellent source of omega-3 fatty acids, which support heart health and reduce inflammation symptoms.
- **Energy and vitality:** Bananas contain potassium and natural carbohydrates for energy that will sustain you throughout the day. This is critical for boosting energy during menopause.
- **Mood support:** Calcium-enriched plant-based milk contributes to bone health and can also positively influence your mood by reducing your risk of hormone-related mineral deficiencies.
- **Extra protein:** If you want to augment this smoothie with a source of complete protein for muscle and metabolic support, just add plant protein powder.

TIP

Add 2 tablespoons of organic plant protein powder if desired (make sure it does not contain thickeners or chemical additives). Hemp protein, pea-rice blends, and lupine flour all contain valuable amino acids.

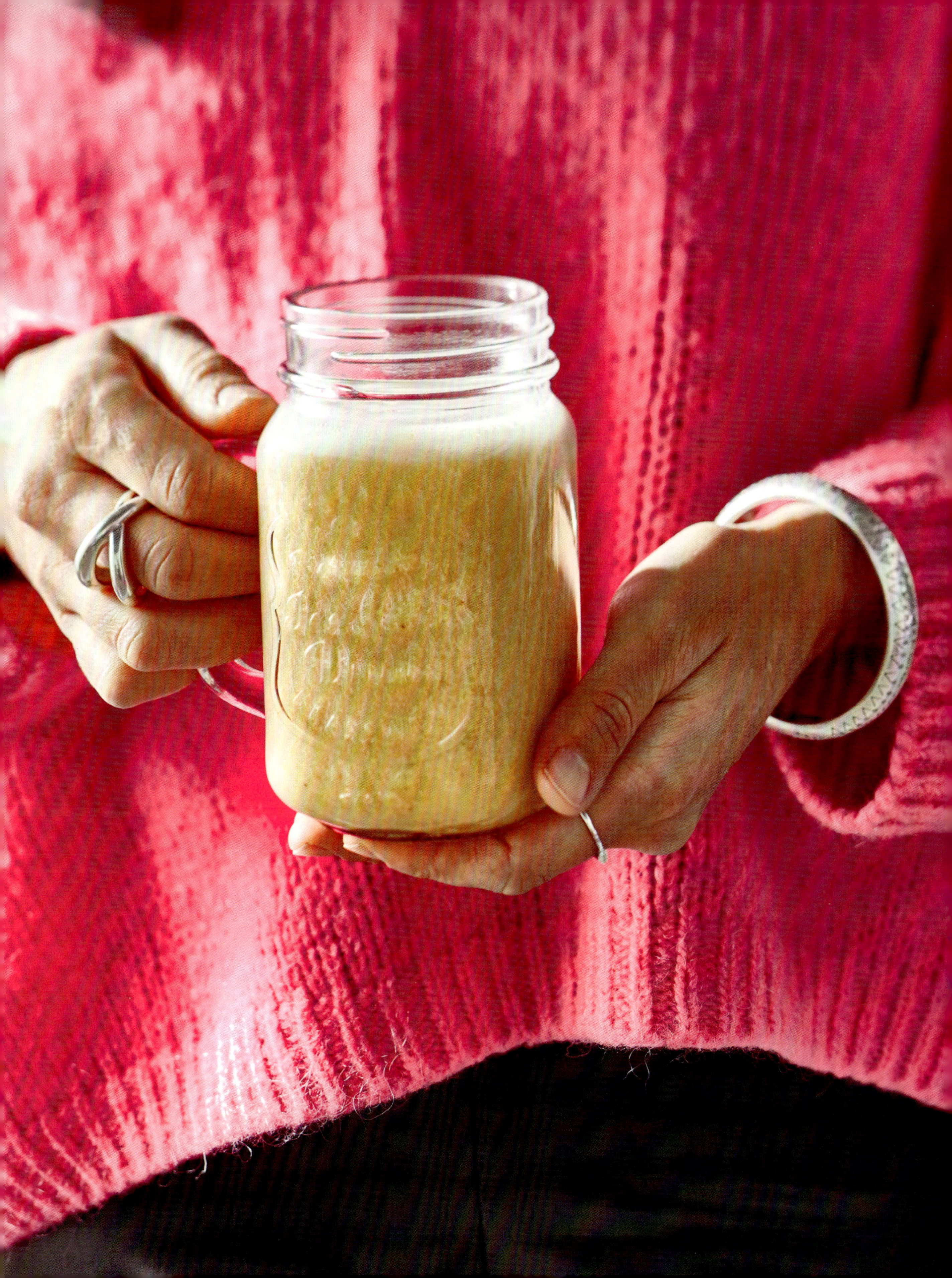

Recipes for Joint Pain and Preventing Osteoporosis

Hormonal changes during menopause may affect bone density and cause joint pain. Foods rich in calcium, vitamin D, and vitamin K are essential for strengthening your bones, relieving inflammation, and ultimately preventing osteoporosis.

Calcium, Vitamin D, and Vitamin K

NUTRITION CLOSE-UP

Calcium

Estrogen hormones play a key role in maintaining bone density and inhibiting bone resorption, which is a natural process of decomposition that releases calcium and other minerals from bone tissue into the blood. The drop in estrogen levels during menopause increases the risk of bone density loss and osteoporosis.

Calcium is a major bone component that contributes to bone structure and strength. Getting enough calcium is essential for maintaining bone density and reducing the risk of fractures.

Calcium also plays a role in preventing dental problems, maintaining good muscle function, regulating communication between nerves and muscles, and reinforcing overall nervous system function. It promotes healthy blood pressure, a robust metabolism, and weight management.

Eating a balanced and varied diet every day will help you meet your calcium needs.

Foods High in Calcium

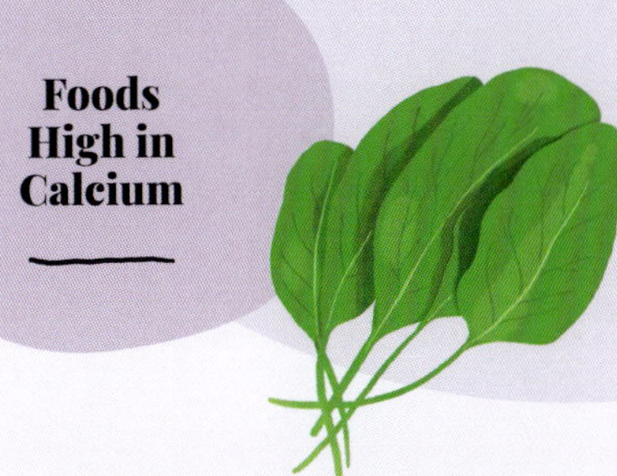

Leafy green vegetables
Broccoli, cabbage, kale, spinach, Swiss chard, lettuce, arugula, lamb's lettuce

Soaked legumes
Beans (white, red, black, cranberry, pinto, mung, adzuki, soy, flageolet, fava), chickpeas, split peas, yellow peas

Fruit
Oranges, fresh and dried figs

Cheese
Pecorino (hard sheep's cheese), Comté

Fatty fish in olive oil
(eat the little ones with the bones—that's where the calcium is!)
Sardine, mackerel, herring, wild salmon, wild tuna

Nuts and seeds
Almonds, chia seeds, sesame seeds

Dairy products
See the following page

Other
Thyme, cinnamon, seaweed (kelp, wakame, royal kombu), shrimp, tofu

What should I know about dairy products and calcium?

Industrially farmed cows release a portion of the antibiotics and hormones they have been given into their milk. Instead of being allowed to feed exclusively on grass, they are given a blend of grasses and grains, which increases the amount of pro-inflammatory omega-6s in the milk and reduces levels of anti-inflammatory omega-3s. To make things worse, the process of pasteurization modifies the proteins in milk and makes them difficult to digest. Only 30 percent of the calcium in conventional dairy products can be absorbed by the body. Luckily, the calcium found in plant foods is much easier for the body to assimilate.

This does not mean you should exclude dairy products from your diet—just make sure you're choosing ones that are high quality. Take a look at the tips on page 108.

Vitamins D and K

Vitamin D facilitates calcium absorption from the intestine to the blood. If you aren't getting enough vitamin D, your body cannot absorb the calcium in the foods you eat even if you are including enough calcium in your diet. As mentioned earlier, good calcium absorption is crucial during menopause for maintaining bone density and preventing osteoporosis.

Vitamin D also plays a role in muscle function and helps prevent muscle pain and weakness. It strengthens the immune system, helps protect the body from infection, regulates mood, and prevents depression.

Vitamin K directs calcium from the blood to the bones and works in tandem with vitamin D to support bone health. It also activates the proteins necessary for blood clot formation to prevent excessive bleeding. In addition, vitamin K helps prevent aortic calcification by activating proteins that ward off calcium deposits in our blood vessels.

Foods High in Vitamins D and K

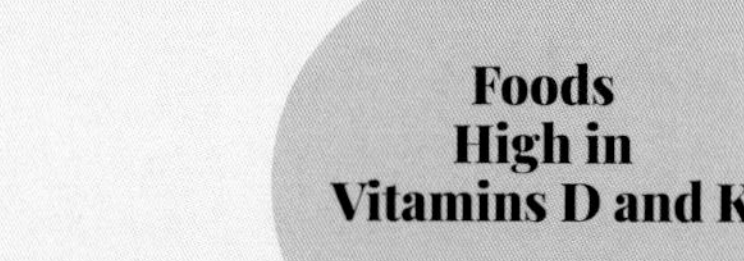

Vitamin D

Fatty fish

Sardines, mackerel, wild salmon, herring, wild tuna, anchovies, trout

Cod liver oil

Eggs

(soft-boiled, sunny-side up, or hard-boiled)

Exposure to the sun*

*Not a food, but thirty minutes a day in short sleeves will give you great exposure. In the summer, try to get your sun exposure in the morning and late afternoon. Sitting or lying in the sun for a significant length of time is dangerous.

Vitamin K

Leafy green vegetables

Broccoli, cabbage, kale, spinach, Swiss chard, lettuce, arugula, lamb's lettuce

Fermented dairy products

Kefir, yogurt, certain cheeses

Bone Broth

Bone broth is rich in collagen and glutamine—both of which are found in animal bone and connective tissue—and this makes it a must during menopause. This broth nourishes the skin, nails, hair, and connective tissue. It also replenishes the body's minerals with trace elements like phosphorus, calcium, magnesium, and silicon. The glutamine in bone broth can soothe intestinal inflammation and repair the lining of your gut. Amino acids like glycine, proline, glucosamine, and chondroitin are wonderful for healing intestinal permeability and preventing problems like osteoarthritis and rheumatoid arthritis.

Makes 1 gallon (4 liters)
Prep: 30 minutes
Cook: 7 hours
Storage: 5 days in the refrigerator

3.3 pounds (1.5 kg) grass-fed beef bones or leftover chicken carcass (with feet)

3 tablespoons apple cider vinegar

4 garlic cloves, crushed

1 onion, peeled

1 carrot, peeled

1 celery stalk

1 handful fresh or dried seaweed

1 tablespoon salt

Your choice of spices (bay leaf, star anise, ginger, turmeric, cinnamon . . .)

Tamari

Salt and pepper

RECIPE

Place all of the ingredients in a large stockpot with 1 gallon (4 liters) of cold water. Bring to a boil then reduce the heat to let it simmer gently for 7 hours. Add water as necessary to keep the bones submerged. Let cool and filter the broth. Correct seasoning as needed with tamari, salt, and pepper.

HOW IT HELPS YOUR BODY

- **Collagen:** The bones and cartilage used in the broth are an excellent source of collagen, which is important for maintaining healthy joints, skin, and hair. Collagen can also help improve skin elasticity and reduce wrinkles.
- **Minerals:** Simmering the bones in water and apple cider vinegar releases minerals like calcium, magnesium, and phosphorous into the broth. These minerals are essential for bone health especially during menopause when the risk of osteoporosis increases.
- **Amino acids:** The amino acids in bone broth, like proline and glycine, are important for tissue repair, digestive health, and reducing inflammation. They may also contribute to better sleep quality by promoting the production of calming neurotransmitters.
- **Antioxidants:** Spices like ginger, turmeric, and cinnamon contain antioxidants and anti-inflammatory compounds. They help reduce oxidative stress and inflammation.
- **Hydration and digestive support:** Bone broth is hydrating and supports healthy digestion by soothing and repairing damage to the gut. Good hydration and optimal digestion are essential for overall wellness.

TIP

Bone broth can be used in soups, to cook rice or quinoa, or consumed as is. You can freeze it in ice cube trays to use later. A layer of fat will form on the top—just stir it into the broth or use it to cook something else!

Miso Soup

This easy-to-digest recipe is great when you want to give your digestive system a break. During menopause, make a point every once in a while to let these organs rest. This makes the liver's work a little easier and improves sleep quality. You can eat this soup anytime—even for breakfast—either by itself or with rice.

Serves 4
Soak: 10 minutes
Prep: 10 minutes
Cook: 10 minutes

2 tablespoons dried seaweed

1 quart (1 liter) dashi

3.5 ounces (100 g) mushrooms (shiitake, oyster mushrooms, enoki mushrooms . . .)

8.8 ounces (250 g) firm tofu

3 tablespoons brown or white miso paste

2 green onions

RECIPE

Place the seaweed in a bowl of cold water and soak for 5 to 10 minutes until rehydrated. Strain and then chop into smaller pieces if necessary.

Bring the dashi broth to a boil in a large pot. Thinly slice the mushrooms and add to the pot. Let them cook for around 5 minutes. Dice the tofu and add to the pot along with the seaweed. Cook for around 2 minutes.

Lower the heat so the broth is just below boiling. Add the miso paste and stir well to dissolve it without creating lumps. Once the miso paste has dissolved, add chopped green onions and serve immediately.

HOW IT HELPS YOUR BODY

- **Isoflavones:** Miso paste is made from fermented soybeans and contains isoflavones. These phytoestrogens imitate the work that estrogen normally does in the body and can help alleviate certain menopause symptoms like hot flashes by balancing hormone levels.
- **Protein:** Tofu is an excellent source of plant protein, which is so important for maintaining muscle mass and a healthy weight. Protein also helps stabilize blood sugar levels to keep your energy up throughout the day.
- **Vitamins B and D:** Mushrooms (especially shiitake and oyster mushrooms) contain vitamins B and D. B vitamins are important for energy metabolism and stress management while vitamin D helps maintain bone health and mood balance.
- **Minerals:** The seaweed in the broth provides minerals like calcium, potassium, and iron that are essential for maintaining cardiovascular health and bodily functions.
- **Hydration:** Dashi broth hydrates the body. This encourages healthy skin and improves dryness symptoms.

Dashi broth

Makes 4 servings
Prep: 15 minutes
Cook: 30 minutes

0.35 ounces (10 g) dried shiitake

0.35 ounces (10 g) dried kombu

RECIPE

Place the shiitake and kombu (cut in half) in a large jar. Pour over 1 quart (1 liter) of boiling water, seal the jar, and let the mixture infuse for 1 to 2 hours or overnight in the refrigerator. Strain and keep for 2 to 3 days in the refrigerator.

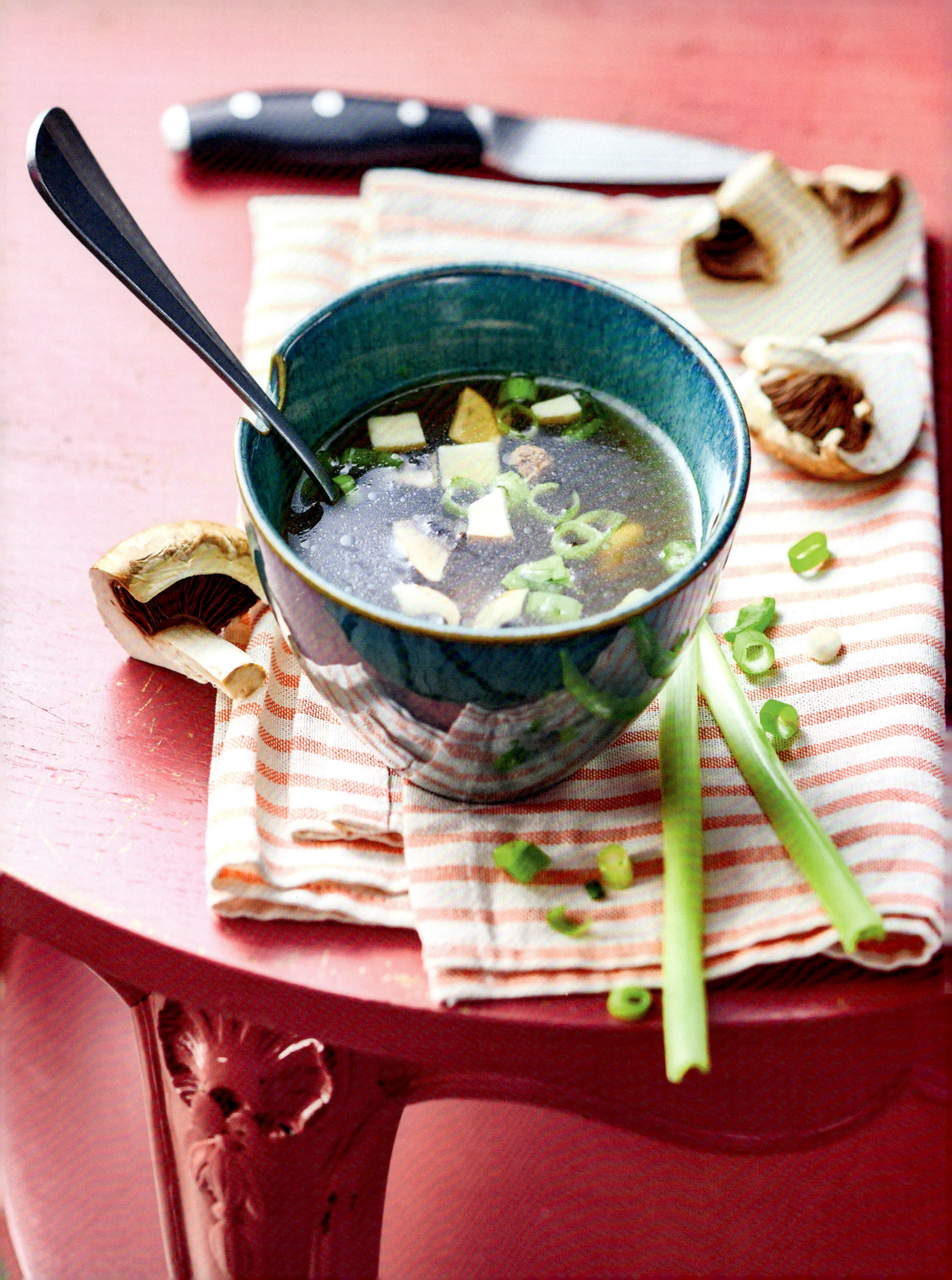

Pho

Pho is a delicious Vietnamese soup traditionally made with beef broth, rice noodles, and aromatic herbs. For this version, we'll use ingredients that are rich in essential nutrients to support well-being during menopause.

Serves 4
Prep: 20 minutes
Cook: 45 minutes

For the broth:

1 onion

2-inch (5 cm) piece fresh ginger

3 garlic cloves

1 tablespoon avocado or olive oil

1.5 quarts (1.5 l) chicken or vegetable broth (homemade if possible)

1 cinnamon stick

3 star anise

4 cloves

1 tablespoon fennel seeds

1 tablespoon tamari

1 tablespoon apple cider vinegar

For the soup:

7 ounces (200 g) whole-grain rice noodles (or buckwheat noodles)

7 ounces (200 g) firm tofu

Olive oil

1 carrot

1 zucchini

7 ounces (200 g) shiitake (fresh or rehydrated)

3.5 ounces (100 g) spinach leaves

3.5 ounces (100 g) mung bean sprouts

2 green onions

1 small bunch fresh cilantro

1 small bunch Thai basil

1 lime

RECIPE

Peel the onion and cut it in half. Grate the ginger, crush the garlic cloves, and sauté everything together in oil for 3 to 4 minutes over medium heat in a large pot to release all of the flavors.

Add the broth and spices to the pot. Bring to a boil, then reduce the heat and let simmer for 30 minutes. Add the tamari and vinegar. Stir well.

While the broth is simmering, cook and drain the noodles following the instructions on the packet.

Dice the tofu. Heat a drizzle of olive oil in a pan and brown the tofu for 5 to 7 minutes until crispy.

Filter the broth and return it to the pot. Cut the carrot and zucchini into thin slivers and thinly slice the shiitake. Add to the pot and cook for 5 minutes until the vegetables are tender.

Add the spinach and let the leaves wilt in the hot broth.

Divide the noodles between 4 large bowls. Sprinkle the tofu on top and pour in the hot broth and vegetables. Garnish with mung bean sprouts along with chopped green onion and herbs. Serve with lime wedges for squeezing.

HOW IT HELPS YOUR BODY

- **Phytoestrogens:** Tofu and mung bean sprouts contain phytoestrogens that help restore hormonal balance.
- **Calcium and magnesium:** Spinach is rich in calcium and magnesium, both of which are essential for bone health.
- **Plant protein:** Tofu is a good source of protein, which is important for maintaining muscle mass.
- **Vitamin D and fiber:** Shiitake mushrooms are rich in fiber and vitamin D, which means they are good for both digestive and immune health.
- **Antioxidants:** Fresh herbs like cilantro and Thai basil are rich in antioxidants that help battle oxidative stress.

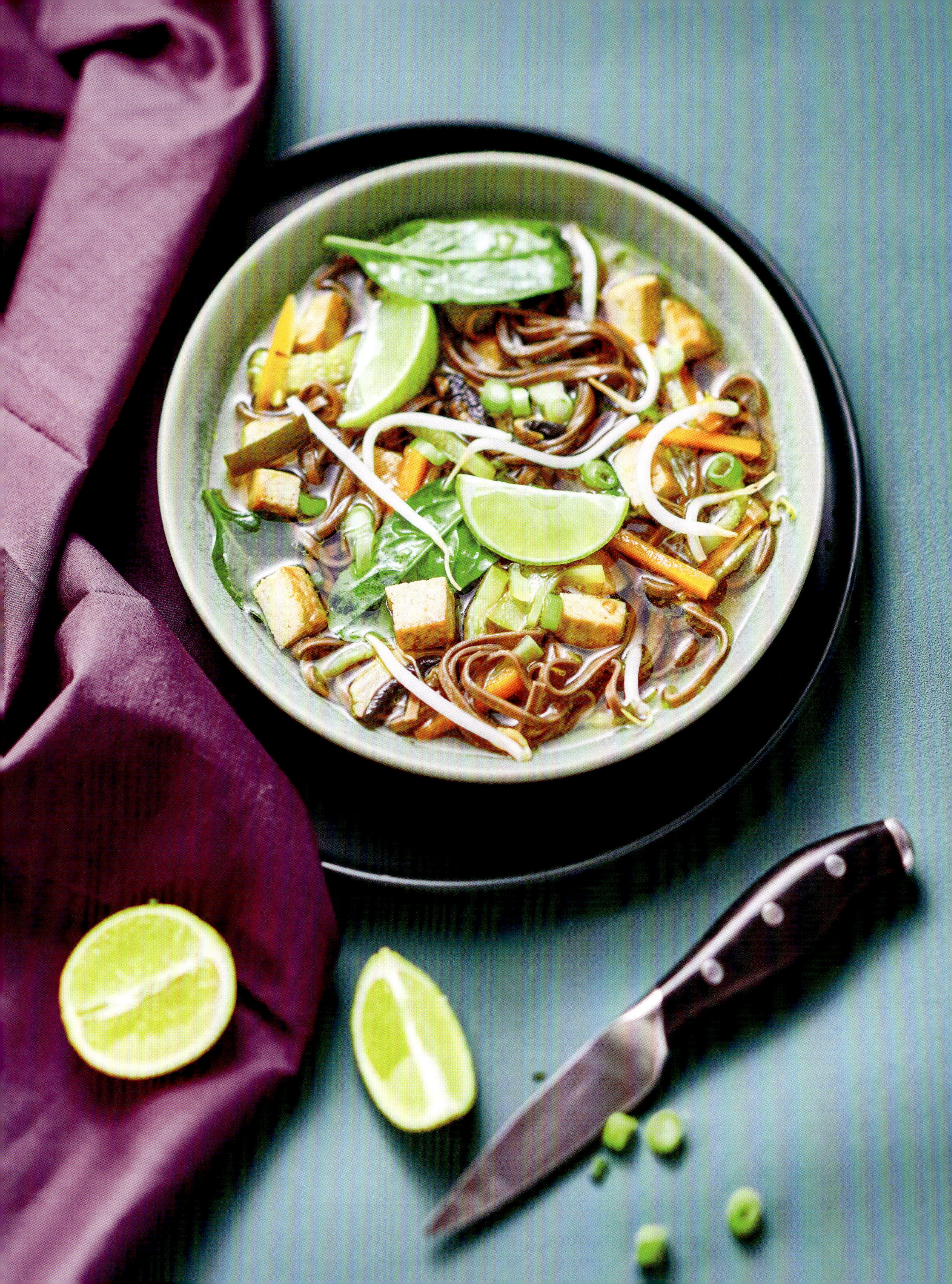

Butternut Squash Soup with Lentils, Turmeric, and Ginger

Serves 4
Prep: 20 minutes
Cook: 35 minutes

1 butternut squash (around 1¾ pounds (800 g))

7 ounces (200 g) coral lentils

1 onion

3 garlic cloves

2-inch (5 cm) piece fresh ginger

2 tablespoons olive oil

1 tablespoon ground turmeric

1 quart (1 l) vegetable broth (homemade if possible)

13.5 fluid ounces (400 ml) coconut milk

Salt and pepper

1 tablespoon pumpkin seeds (optional)

1 small bunch fresh cilantro (optional)

RECIPE

Peel the butternut squash and cut into cubes. Rinse the lentils under cold water until the water runs clear. Peel the onion and garlic. Thinly slice the onion and mince the garlic. Grate the ginger.

Heat the oil over medium heat in a large pot and sauté the onion until translucent (around 5 minutes). Add the garlic and ginger. Cook for another 2 minutes. Add the squash cubes and the turmeric and stir everything together. Pour in the broth and bring to a boil.

Add the lentils, lower the heat, and let cook for 20 minutes until the squash and lentils are tender. Use an immersion blender to blend the soup until smooth (you can also use a regular blender if you prefer—blend it a little at a time if you need to). Stir in the coconut milk. Season with salt and pepper and cook for 5 more minutes to allow the flavors to develop.

Serve the soup hot. Sprinkle each bowl with pumpkin seeds and chopped cilantro.

HOW IT HELPS YOUR BODY

- **Nutrients:** Butternut squash is rich in vitamins A and C, fiber, and antioxidants. Coral lentils provide plant protein and fiber for healthy muscle mass and digestion.
- **Anti-inflammatory properties:** Turmeric contains a powerful natural anti-inflammatory called curcumin. Adding ginger, which is rich in gingerol, activates the curcumin to maximize its health benefits.
- **Hydration and healthy fats:** Coconut milk contains healthy fatty acids and contributes to hydration, healthy skin, and reduced inflammation.
- **Digestive support:** Ginger is renowned for its digestive benefits. It is particularly helpful for relieving nausea and other stomach discomfort.

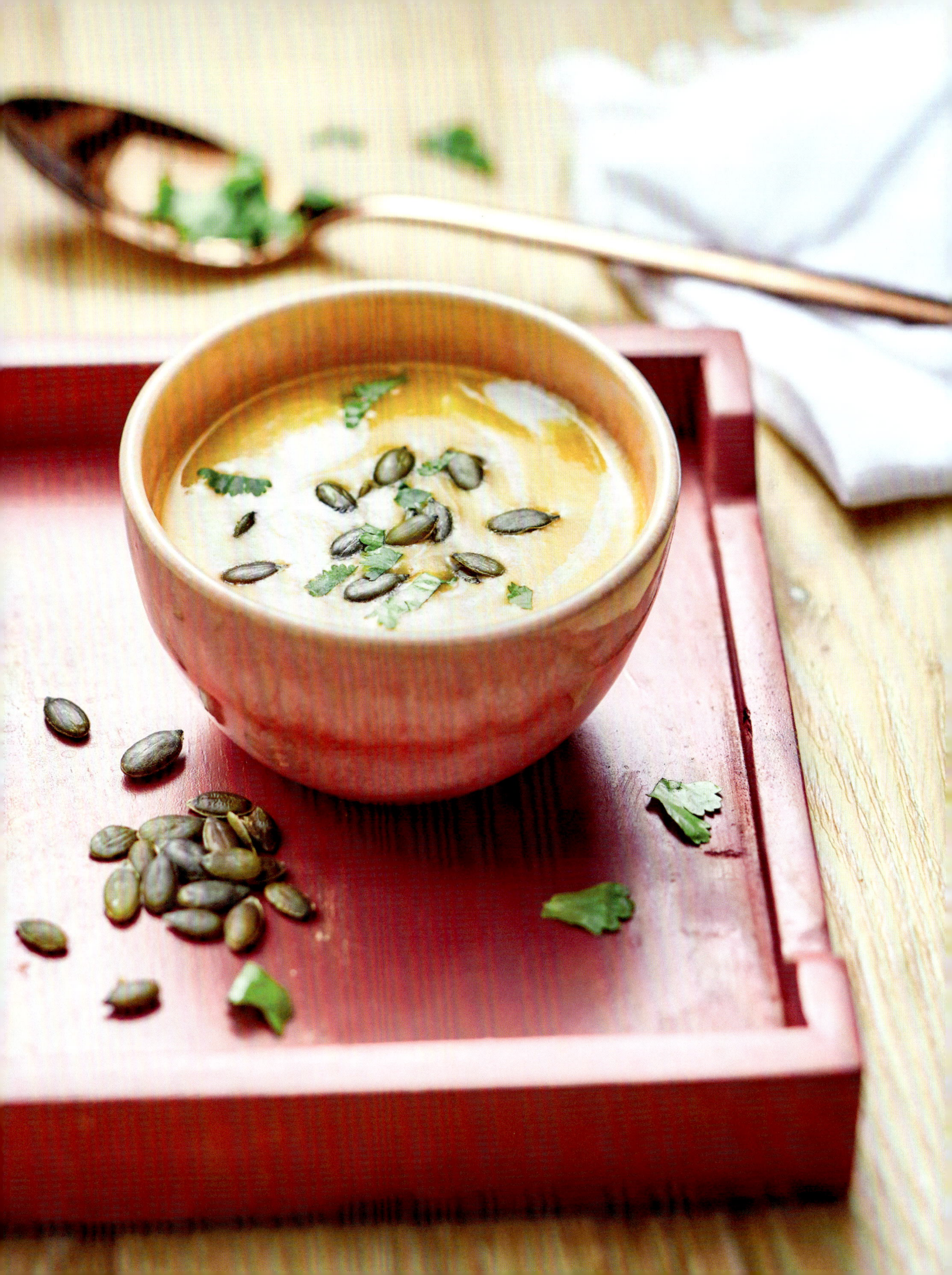

Roasted Sweet Potato Tartines

Serves 4
Prep: 20 minutes
Cook: 25 minutes

2 large sweet potatoes
2 tablespoons olive oil
Salt and pepper
2 avocados
Juice of 1 lemon
6 radishes
1 cucumber
1 small bunch fresh cilantro
1 handful pumpkin seeds
3.5 ounces (100 g) feta

RECIPE

Preheat the oven to 400°F (200°C).

Wash the sweet potatoes and slice lengthwise into ½-inch- (1 cm-) thick pieces. Transfer to a baking sheet lined with parchment paper. Drizzle with oil on both sides and season with salt and pepper. Bake for 25 minutes until the sweet potatoes are tender and golden (turn over halfway through for even cooking).

Crush the avocados in a bowl and add the lemon juice, salt, and pepper. Stir well. Thinly slice the radishes and cucumber. Chop the cilantro.

Once the sweet potato slices are cooked, remove them from the oven and spread a generous layer of the crushed avocado mixture on top of each one. Add the radish and cucumber slices and sprinkle with pumpkin seeds and cilantro.

Crumble the feta over the top for extra creaminess and salty flavor. Serve immediately.

HOW IT HELPS YOUR BODY

- **Nutrients:** Sweet potatoes are an excellent source of vitamins A and C as well as fiber. These help support healthy digestion and skin.
- **Hormonal support:** Avocados are rich in vitamin E and monounsaturated fatty acids that help balance hormones.
- **Anti-inflammatory properties:** Cucumber and radish provide antioxidants and anti-inflammatory compounds.
- **Magnesium and zinc:** Pumpkin seeds are rich in magnesium and zinc. These two minerals are essential for hormone and bone health.
- **Hydration and staying cool:** Cucumber and lemon offer the body welcome hydration and refreshment.

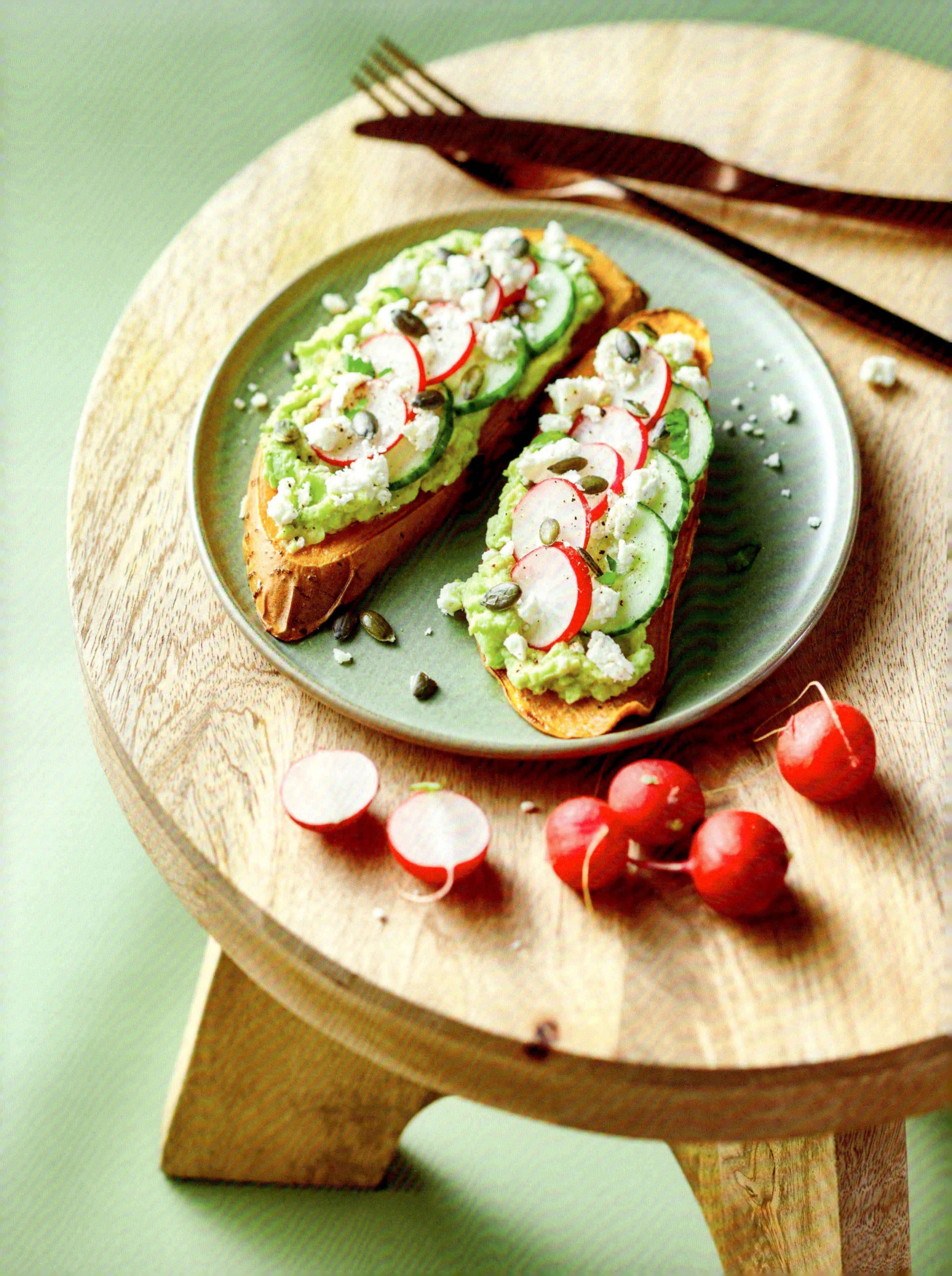

Smoked Herring and Potato Salad

Serves 4
Prep: 20 minutes
Cook: 20 minutes

1.3 pounds (600 g) potatoes

7 ounces (200 g) smoked herring fillets

1 red onion

2 cornichon pickles

1 apple

3 teaspoons plain yogurt (raw sheep or goat's milk)

2 tablespoons whole-grain mustard

1 tablespoon apple cider vinegar

2 tablespoons olive oil

Salt and pepper

1 small bunch chives

1 small bunch fresh dill

RECIPE

Wash the potatoes. Transfer to a large pot and cover with cold salted water. Bring to a boil. Reduce the heat and let cook 15 to 20 minutes until tender. Drain and peel the potatoes if necessary before cutting into cubes.

Cut the herring fillets into medium-size pieces. Peel and thinly slice the red onion. Cut the pickles into rounds and dice the apple.

Combine the yogurt, mustard, vinegar, and oil. Season with salt and pepper.

Combine the potato cubes with the herring, onion, pickles, and apple in a large bowl. Pour in the vinaigrette and gently toss. Chop the chives and dill, add them to the bowl, and toss again. Serve immediately or refrigerate for 1 hour to let the flavors intermingle.

HOW IT HELPS YOUR BODY

Omega-3 fatty acids: Herring is an excellent source of omega-3 fatty acids, which are beneficial for cardiovascular health and can also help reduce inflammation.

Protein and minerals: Herring and potatoes contain a hefty amount of protein and minerals like potassium and magnesium that are essential for muscle and bone health.

Fiber and vitamins: Potatoes and apples provide fiber, which promotes healthy digestion, as well as vitamins C and B6. These are important for the immune system and managing stress.

Probiotics: Yogurt made with raw sheep or goat's milk contains probiotics that are good for your gut. Since hormonal changes can often have a negative effect on gut health, menopause is an important time to include probiotics in your cooking.

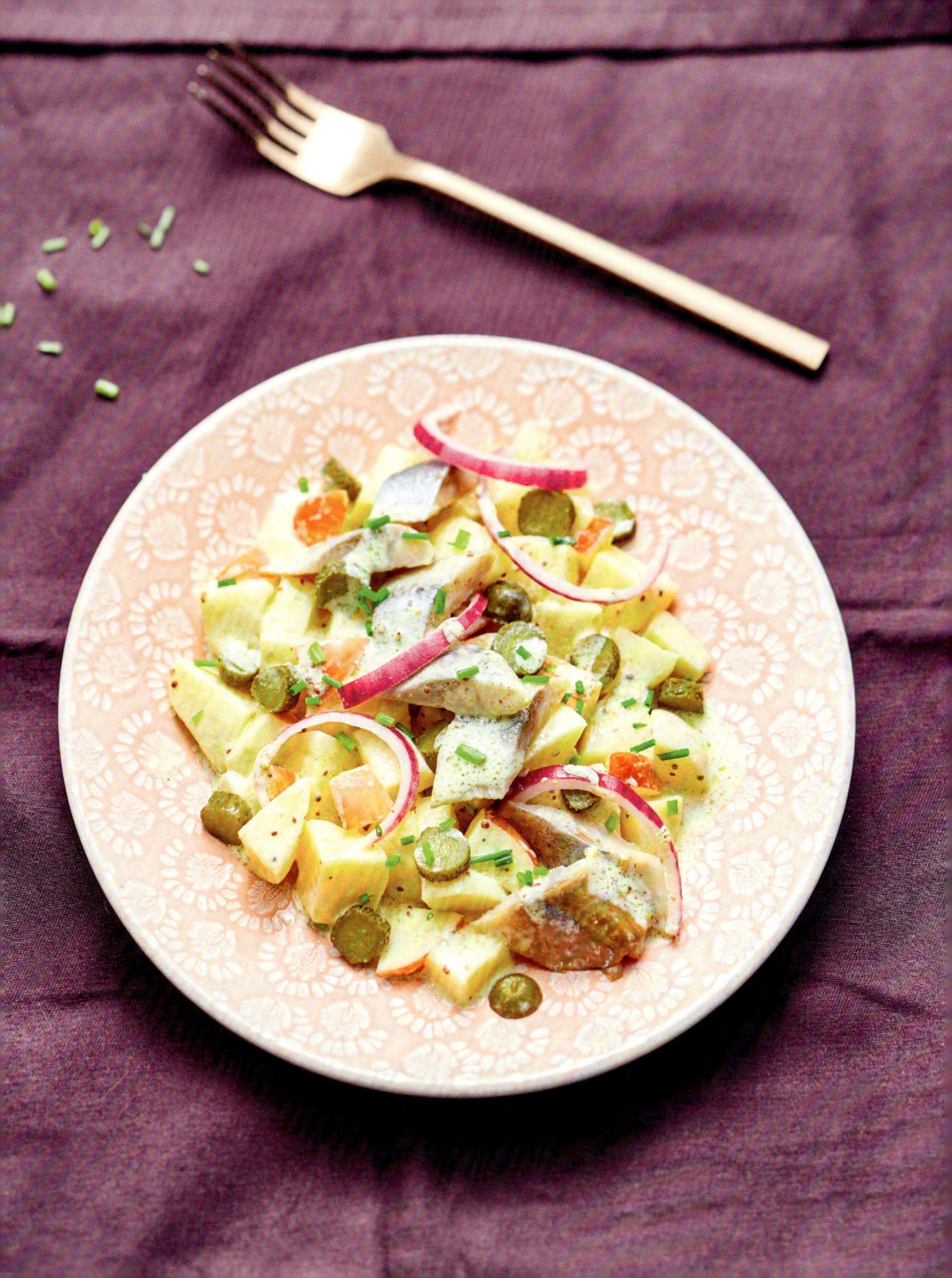

Green on Green Salad

Serves 4
Prep: 20 minutes

7 ounces (200 g) kale

Juice of 1 lemon, divided

3 tablespoons olive oil, divided

5.3 ounces (150 g) firm tofu

1 avocado

1 cucumber

2 celery stalks

1 tablespoon apple cider vinegar

1 tablespoon tamari

Salt and pepper

7 ounces (200 g) spinach leaves

7 ounces (200 g) cooked chickpeas (or 1 can of chickpeas, drained)

1.76 ounces (50 g) pumpkin seeds

1.76 ounces (50 g) cooked quinoa (optional)

2 ounces (60 g) pecorino, grated or shaved

RECIPE

Remove any tough kale stems and chop the leaves. Transfer to a bowl and add a drizzle of lemon juice and 1 tablespoon oil. Massage the kale with your hands for 2 to 3 minutes until tender.

Cut the tofu into cubes. Cut the avocado in half, remove the pit, and slice the flesh. Dice the cucumber and celery.

Combine the remaining lemon juice and oil with the vinegar and tamari. Season with salt and pepper.

To the bowl of kale, add the spinach, tofu, chickpeas, cucumber, celery, pumpkin seeds, and quinoa, if using. Pour in the vinaigrette and toss.

Arrange the avocado slices on top of the salad. Top with pecorino and serve immediately.

HOW IT HELPS YOUR BODY

- **Protein and amino acids:** Tofu and chickpeas provide high-quality protein that is essential for maintaining muscle mass and overall well-being.
- **Antioxidants and fiber:** Kale and spinach are rich in antioxidants and fiber. This means they are good for digestion and help fight against free radicals.
- **Pumpkin seeds:** Rich in magnesium and zinc, pumpkin seeds are excellent for bone health and immune function.
- **Healthy fats:** Avocados and olive oil contain monounsaturated fatty acids that are beneficial for cardiovascular health.
- **Essential micronutrients:** Kale is an excellent source of vitamin K, vitamin C, and calcium, all of which are important for bone health and reducing inflammation.

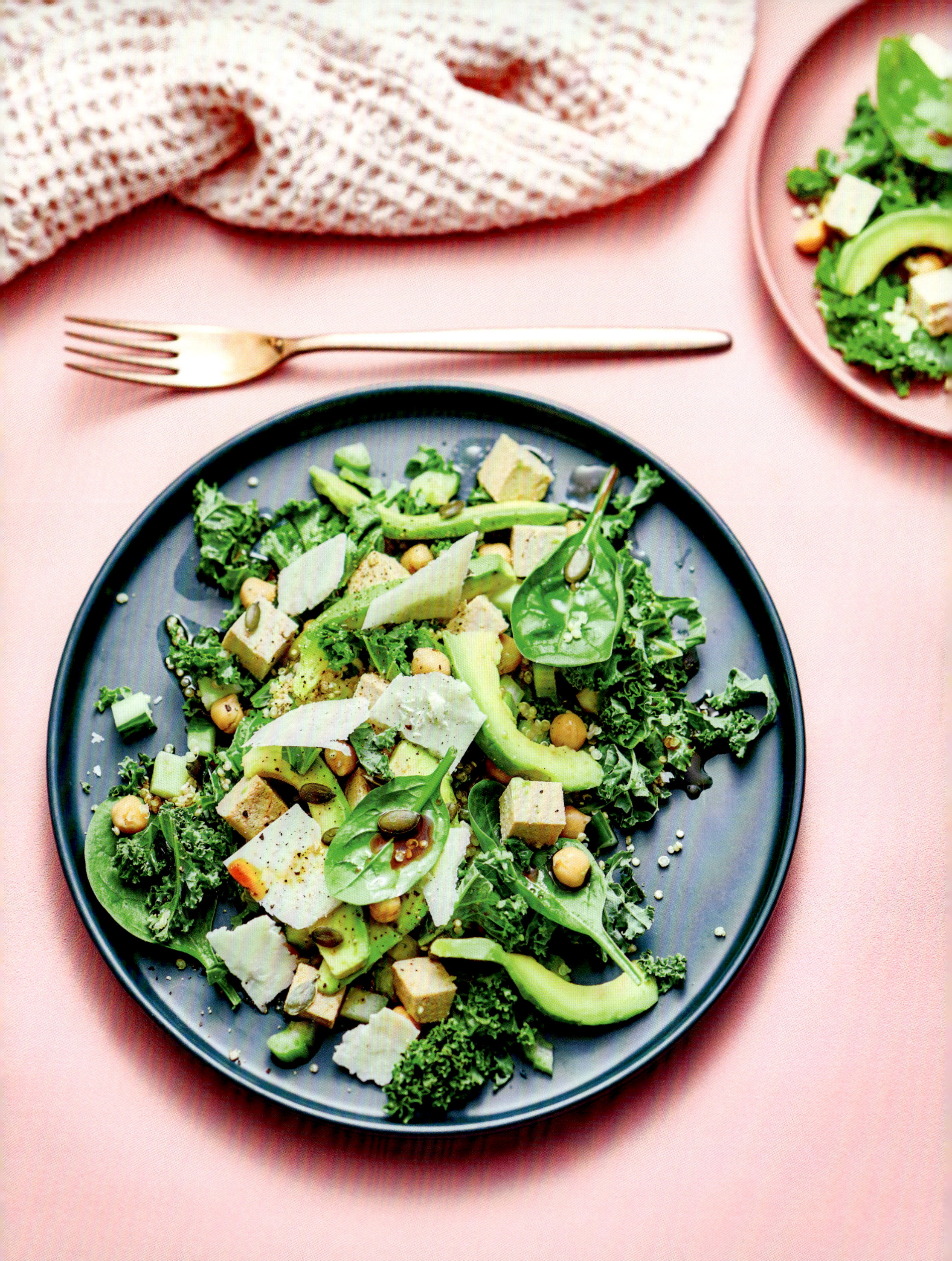

Green Smoothies

Serves 1
Prep: 15 minutes

Detox:

1 ounce (30 g) fresh spinach

½ cucumber (around 2 ounces [60 g])

2 ounces (60 g) fennel

6 sprigs of fresh parsley

1 kiwi, peeled

Juice of ½ lemon

¼ cup/2 fluid ounces (60 ml) coconut water

Energy:

1 ounce (30 g) kale

1 celery stalk

½ green apple*

1 small banana, peeled

¾-inch (2 cm) piece fresh ginger

Juice of ½ lemon

¼ cup/2 fluid ounces (60 ml) water

Antioxidant:

1 ounce (30 g) arugula

1 ounce (30 g) Swiss chard (or spinach)

2.6 ounces (75 g) berries (raspberries, blueberries . . .)

½ ounce (15 g) chia seeds

½ cup/4 fluid ounces (120 ml) almond milk

* Depending on your personal preference, how powerful your blender is, and where your fruit comes from (organic or not), you can peel the apple if you want to.

RECIPE

Add all of the ingredients for the smoothie to a blender and blend until smooth. Enjoy immediately.

HOW IT HELPS YOUR BODY

Essential nutrients: Green smoothies are an excellent source of the vitamins, minerals, and antioxidants that are so needed during menopause. The spinach, cucumber, avocado, fennel, parsley, kale, green apple, banana, ginger, arugula, Swiss chard, berries, and chia seeds in these recipes provide a wide range of nutrients like vitamin C, vitamin K, magnesium, potassium, fiber, and antioxidants.

Reducing inflammation: Green smoothies contain ingredients rich in antioxidants and anti-inflammatory compounds like ginger, berries, and green vegetables.

Hydration and electrolyte balance: Some green smoothies incorporate ingredients like coconut water, which is rich in electrolytes, and hydrating vegetables like cucumber. This helps maintain healthy hydration and electrolyte balance.

Digestive support and hormone balance: The fiber in green vegetables, fruit, and chia seeds promotes healthy digestion and reduces bloating and constipation. Other ingredients like fennel also support hormonal balance and alleviate digestive troubles linked to hormone fluctuations.

Mental and emotional well-being: Green smoothies can also play a role in regulating mood and reducing stress thanks to vitamin B, magnesium, and other nutrients that contribute to nervous system health and neurotransmitter production.

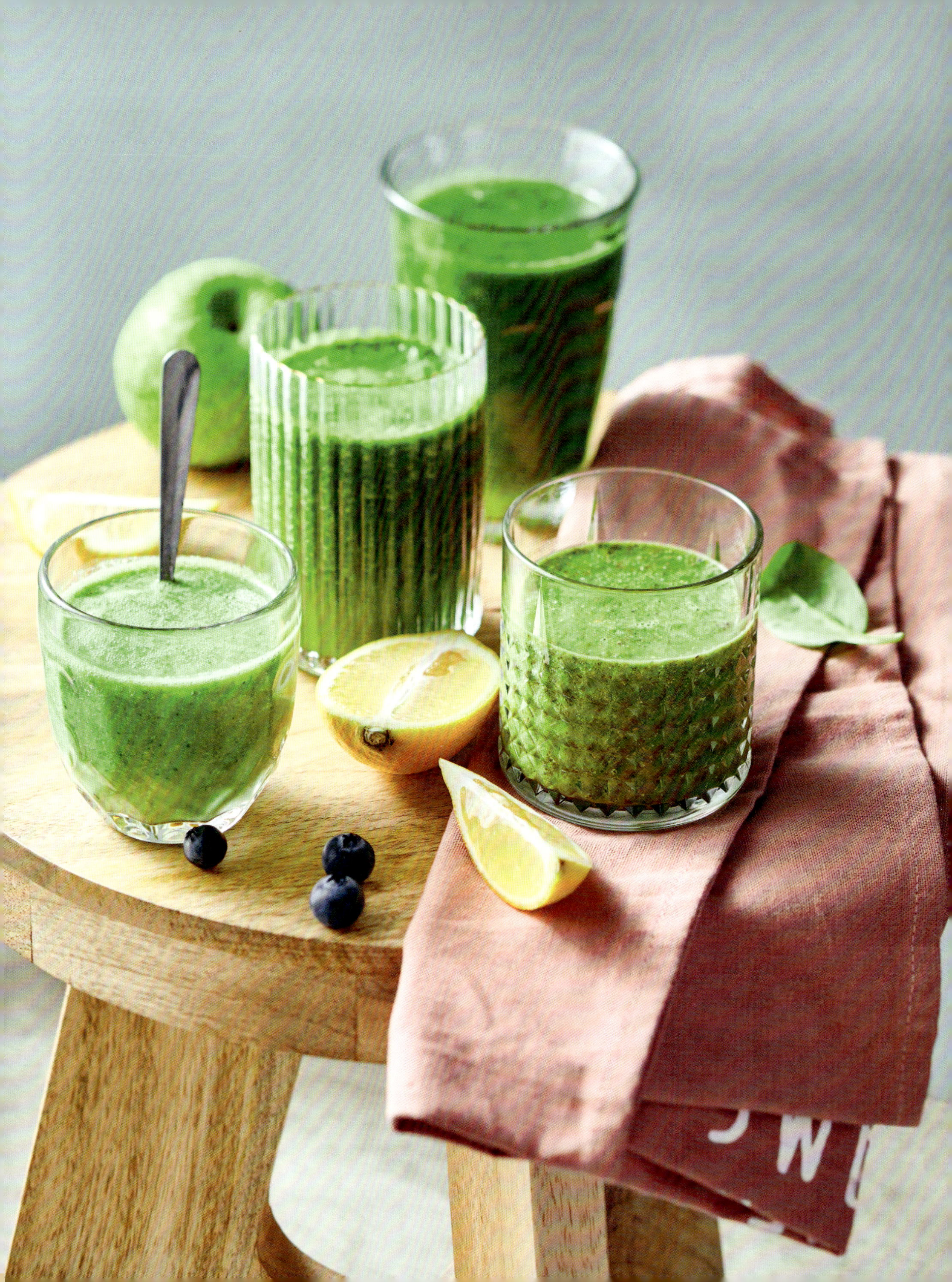

Recipes for Gut Health

Menopause is often accompanied by digestive issues like bloating and a feeling of heaviness in the body. A diet rich in fiber, probiotics, and antioxidants can keep your gut microbiome in balance and improve digestion.

Cooking with Whole Grains

Whole grains are a high-quality source of carbohydrates and are also rich in fiber, nutrients, and minerals that the body needs—especially during premenopause and menopause. In order to reap these benefits, though, you need to know how to prepare whole grains properly (the soaking process will be explained in the following recipes).

Improved bowel function

Whole grains like whole wheat, brown rice, oats, quinoa, and rye are excellent sources of fiber. Fiber plays an essential role in regulating bowel movements and helps prevent constipation, which is something that can become more of an issue during menopause when estrogen levels drop and disrupt gut flora balance. The high fiber content in whole grains promotes good gut health thanks to nondigestible fiber compounds known as prebiotics. Prebiotics nourish the beneficial bacteria (probiotics) in our intestines to foster a balanced gut microbiome.

Better blood sugar levels

The fiber in whole grains increases feelings of satiety, which can help with maintaining a healthy weight. During menopause, the body's metabolism slows down and weight gain happens more easily. The soluble fiber found in whole grains slows down the absorption of sugar into the bloodstream. This makes it easier to manage blood sugar levels and is particularly helpful for menopausal women since hormone fluctuations may impact insulin sensitivity.

Overall well-being and energy

Whole grains are rich in vitamins (like B vitamins, which are important for energy metabolism) and minerals (like magnesium, iron, and zinc). These nutrients are essential for overall wellness and can help reduce certain menopause symptoms like fatigue and mood swings.

Bone health

Whole grains also contain important bone health minerals like magnesium and phosphorus. During menopause, the drop in estrogen levels can lead to increased bone loss and a greater risk of developing osteoporosis. A diet rich in these minerals will help maintain bone density.

Barley Salad with Feta and Fresh Vegetables

Serves 4
Soak: 12 hours
Prep: 20 minutes
Cook: 1 hour

7 ounces (200 g) barley groats

7 ounces (200 g) cherry tomatoes

5.3 ounces (150 g) feta

1 bell pepper

½ cucumber

1 red onion

4 tablespoons olive oil

2 tablespoons apple cider vinegar

1 teaspoon dried oregano

Salt and pepper

3.5 ounces (100 g) arugula

4 tablespoons pumpkin seeds

RECIPE

Soaking the barley for 12 hours will reduce the cooking time. When that's finished, transfer the barley to a pot along with 4 times its volume of cold salted water. Bring to a boil and cook for 1 hour over low heat until tender. Drain and let cool.

Cut the cherry tomatoes in half, crumble the feta, dice the pepper and cucumber, and peel and thinly slice the onion. Stir the vegetables into the cooked barley.

Whisk together the oil, vinegar, and oregano. Season with salt and pepper. Pour the vinaigrette over the salad, toss, and top with pumpkin seeds before serving.

HOW IT HELPS YOUR BODY

- **Fiber:** Barley and raw vegetables are rich in fiber, which means they promote healthy digestion and help prevent constipation.
- **Calcium and magnesium:** Feta is a good source of calcium, which is essential for maintaining bone density, and pumpkin seeds provide magnesium to prevent muscle cramps and promote relaxation.
- **Antioxidants:** Cherry tomatoes, bell peppers, and cucumbers are rich in vitamins and antioxidants that reduce oxidative stress and protect the body's cells.
- **Anti-inflammation:** Olive oil contains polyphenols and monounsaturated fatty acids. Both have anti-inflammatory properties.
- **Hormonal balance:** The fiber and nutrients in this salad help regulate hormone levels and improve your overall health during menopause.

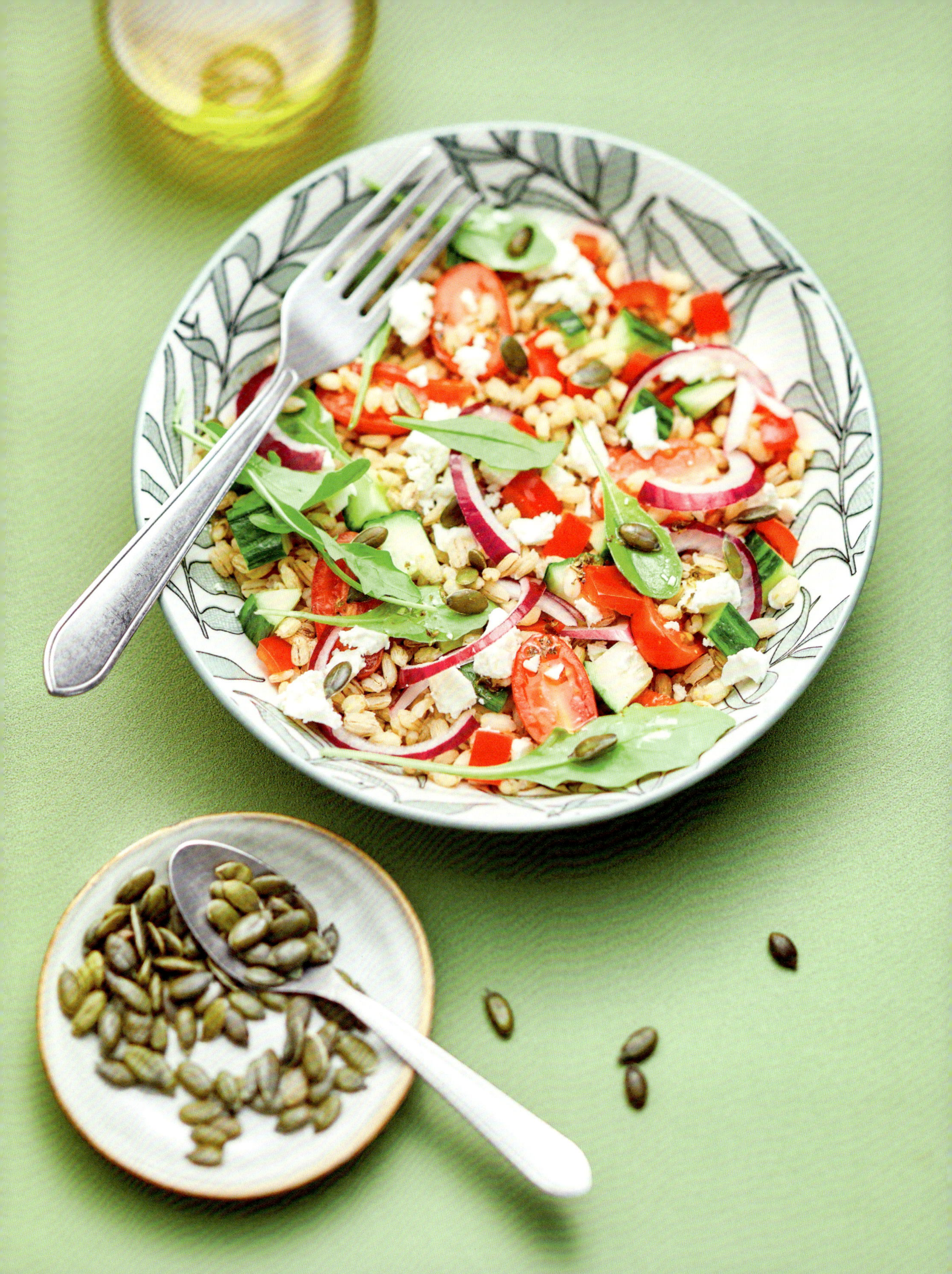

Brown Rice Risotto with Mushrooms

Serves 4
Prep: 15 minutes
Cook: 1 hour

1 onion

2 garlic cloves

17.6 ounces (500 g) mushrooms (button, shiitake, etc.)

1 quart (1 l) vegetable broth

2 tablespoons olive oil, divided

8.8 ounces (250 g) brown rice

1 tablespoon nutritional yeast

1.76 ounces (50 g) Parmesan, grated

Salt and pepper

2 tablespoons fresh parsley

RECIPE

Peel and thinly slice the onion and garlic. Thinly slice the mushrooms.

Heat the broth and keep warm.

In a large pan or pot, heat 1 tablespoon of oil over medium heat. Sauté the onion until translucent (around 5 minutes). Add the garlic and cook for 1 minute. Add the mushrooms, then cook them until they release their liquid and are tender (5 to 7 minutes).

Add the rice and stir together. Toast the rice for 2 to 3 minutes, then add 1 ladleful of broth and stir until the liquid has been absorbed. Continue adding broth, one ladleful at a time, stirring frequently and waiting for each ladleful to be absorbed before adding the next one. This will take around 45 minutes.

When the rice is tender and creamy, add the nutritional yeast and Parmesan. Season with salt and pepper. Add 1 tablespoon of oil and sprinkle with chopped parsley. Serve hot.

HOW IT HELPS YOUR BODY

- **Fiber:** Brown rice and mushrooms are rich in fiber, which regulates digestion and prevents constipation.
- **Magnesium and vitamin D:** Brown rice and mushrooms contain magnesium. Mushrooms also contain vitamin D, which is essential for bone and muscle health.
- **Vitamin B:** The B vitamins in the nutritional yeast are useful for fending off fatigue and supporting brain function.
- **Heart support:** Olive oil contains polyphenols and monounsaturated fatty acids that reduce inflammation and stabilize cholesterol levels.
- **Anti-inflammation and immune support:** The antioxidants in onions and garlic reduce inflammation and strengthen the immune system. The vitamin K in parsley supports blood clotting and bone health.

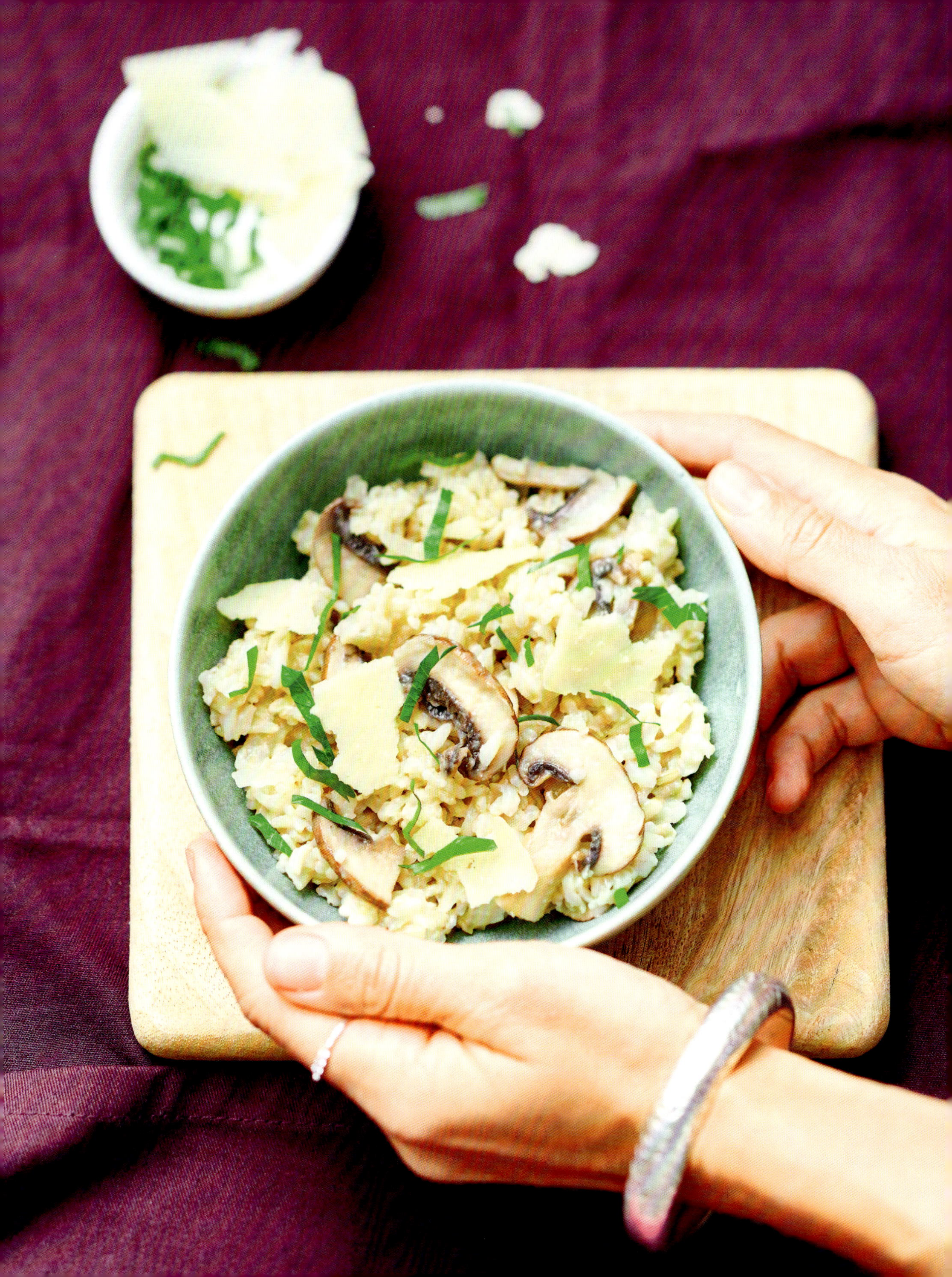

Quinoa Croquettes with Lemon Yogurt Sauce

Serves 4
Prep: 20 minutes
Cook: 45 minutes

5.3 ounces (150 g) quinoa

2 tablespoons olive oil

1 medium onion

2 garlic cloves

7 ounces (200 g) fresh spinach

2 eggs

1.76 ounces (50 g) Parmesan, grated

1.76 ounces (50 g) semi-wholemeal einkorn flour

Zest of 1 lemon

2 tablespoons sesame seeds

Salt and pepper

For the sauce:

7 ounces (200 g) Greek yogurt made with sheep's milk (raw if possible)

Juice of 1 lemon

2 tablespoons chives, chopped

Salt and pepper

RECIPE

Rinse the quinoa under cold water. Cook in a pot of salted boiling water and follow the instructions on the box (roughly 15 minutes). Drain and let cool.

Preheat the oven to 350°F (180°C).

Heat the oil over medium heat in a large pan. Peel and thinly slice the onion and garlic. Add to the pan and cook until translucent. Add the spinach and sauté until wilted.

Combine the quinoa, cooked vegetables, eggs, Parmesan, flour, lemon zest, and sesame seeds. Season with salt and pepper. Use your hands to form small balls or pancake shapes and place on a baking sheet lined with parchment paper.

Bake for 25 to 30 minutes until the croquettes are golden and crispy. Turn them over halfway through baking.

Mix together the sauce ingredients until combined.

Serve these croquettes with a green salad and fresh vegetables.

HOW IT HELPS YOUR BODY

- **Blood sugar regulation:** Quinoa is rich in protein and fiber and helps stabilize blood sugar levels to avoid spikes and sudden drops in blood sugar.
- **Calcium, magnesium, and phosphorous:** Quinoa, Parmesan, and spinach contain minerals that promote bone health and prevent osteoporosis.
- **Anti-inflammation:** Spinach and sesame seeds contain antioxidants and essential fatty acids that help reduce inflammation.
- **Fiber:** Quinoa and spinach are rich in fiber, which promotes regular bowel movements and prevents constipation.
- **Probiotics:** Raw Greek yogurt contains probiotics that support gut health.

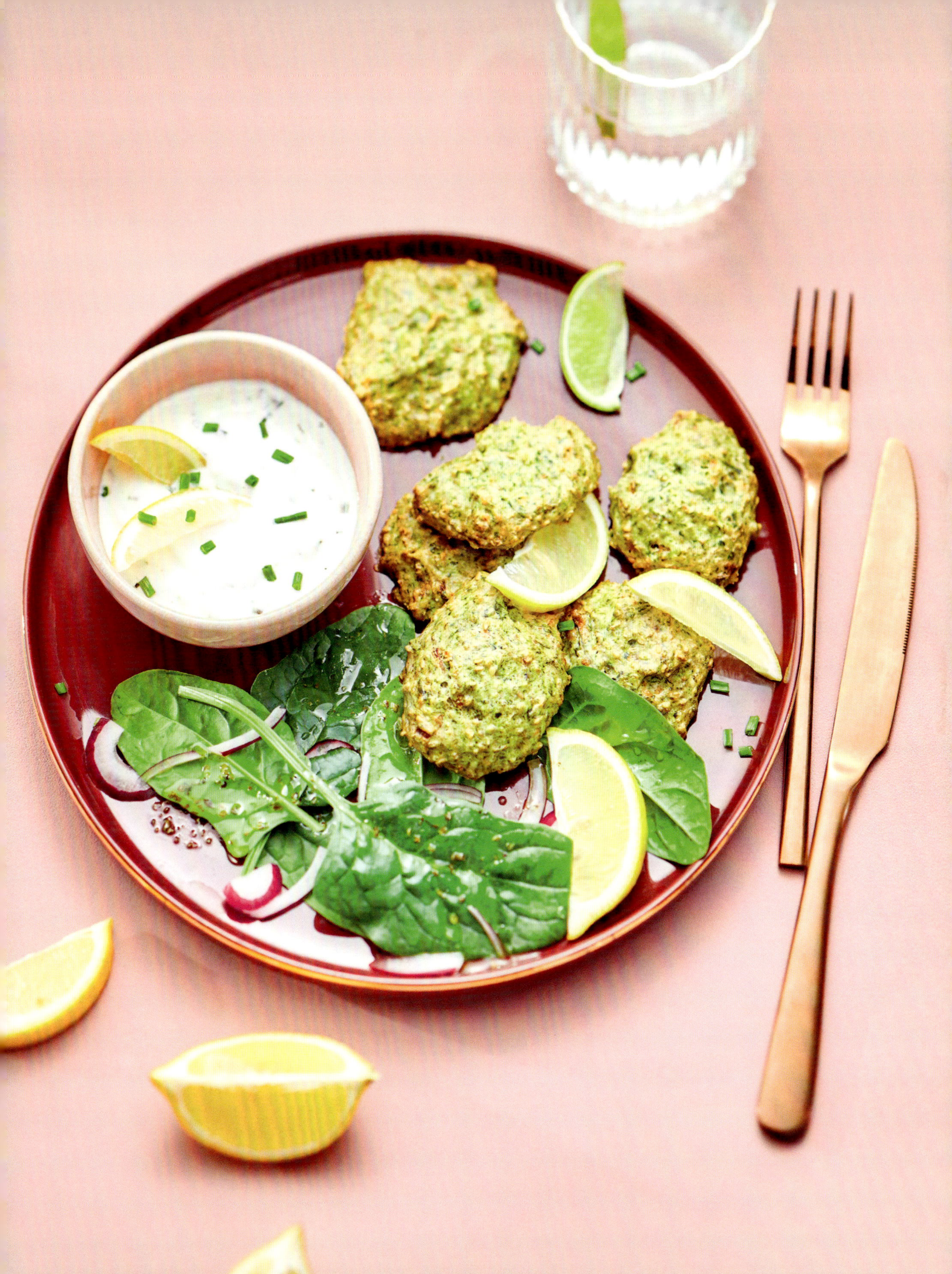

Buckwheat Galettes

Makes 12 galettes
Prep: 20 minutes
Rest: 2 hours
Cook: 40 minutes

11.6 ounces (330 g) buckwheat flour

0.35 ounces (10 g) coarse salt

1 egg

Butter (or ghee)

RECIPE

Combine the flour and salt in a large bowl. Make a well and gradually pour in 3 cups (750 ml) of water. Stir vigorously with a wooden spoon. The batter should be thick but fluid.

Add the egg, which will give the batter a beautiful color when it cooks, and stir well. Let the batter rest under a dish towel for around 2 hours in the refrigerator.

Heat the butter in a pan over low to medium heat. Once the butter is melted, pour 1 ladleful of batter into the pan and quickly tilt it to spread the batter over the entire surface of the pan. Cook each side 1 to 2 minutes. To turn the galette over, use a spatula and lift the edges before quickly flipping it over.

Serve the galettes with the filling of your choice (see ideas on pages 90 and 91).

HOW IT HELPS YOUR BODY

- **B vitamins:** Eggs contain B vitamins, which are useful for energy metabolism and healthy nervous system function. They also support overall energy and well-being.
- **Magnesium:** Buckwheat contains magnesium, which contributes to bone health by promoting bone density and reducing the risk of osteoporosis.
- **Fiber:** Buckwheat flour contains fiber, which improves digestion and prevents constipation caused by hormonal fluctuations.
- **Flavonoids and polyphenols:** Buckwheat contains anti-inflammatory antioxidants that help reduce joint pain and inflammation.
- **Complete protein:** Eggs contain high-quality protein that helps stabilize blood sugar levels and maintain muscle mass during hormonal changes.
- **Healthy fats:** Butter and ghee contain healthy fats that promote satiety to help regulate blood sugar and provide essential fatty acids that are necessary for healthy hormone and cell function.

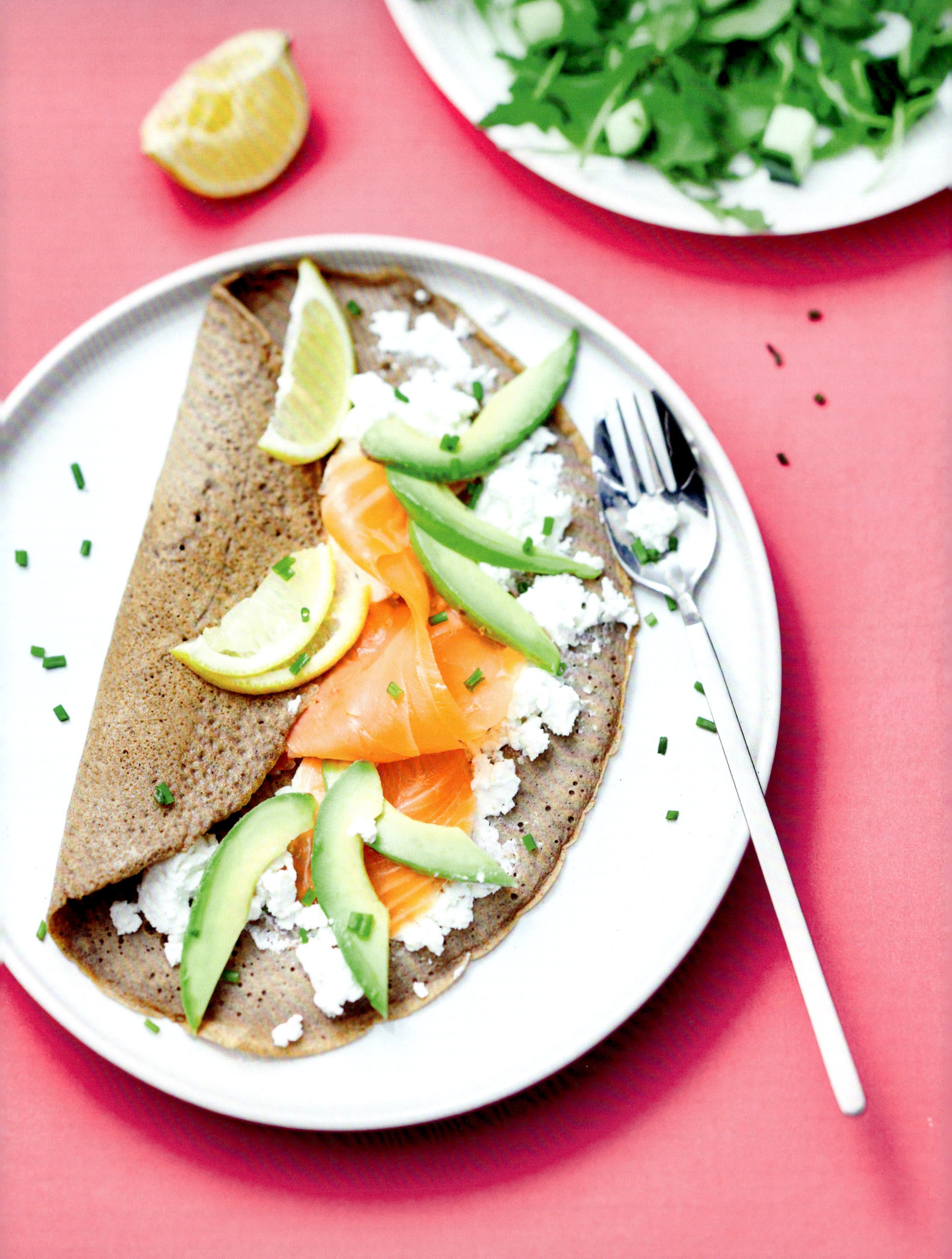

Filling Ideas

Mushrooms, caramelized onions, and Comté

Serves 1
Prep: 10 minutes
Cook: 10 minutes

1 tablespoon olive oil

1 small onion, sliced

1.76 ounces (50 g) button mushrooms, sliced

1 tablespoon balsamic vinegar

1 ounce (30 g) grated Comté

Salt and pepper

Heat the olive oil in a pan to cook the sliced onion and mushrooms until the mushrooms release their liquid. Deglaze the pan with balsamic vinegar and cook until it has evaporated.

Place the galette in a hot oiled pan. Add the onion and mushroom mixture along with the cheese. Fold over the edges of the galette and cook for 5 minutes until the cheese starts to melt. Season with salt and pepper and serve.

HELPFUL INGREDIENTS

Mushrooms: are a source of vitamin D, promote calcium absorption, and support bone health.

Onions: contain antioxidants that help reduce inflammation and support the immune system.

Comté: this cheese is rich in calcium (to support bone health), protein (to maintain muscle mass), and probiotics (to nourish gut flora).

Ratatouille and goat cheese

Serves 1
Prep: 15 minutes
Cook: 10 minutes

1.76 ounces (50 g) homemade ratatouille (eggplant, zucchini, bell pepper, tomato, onion, garlic, herbes de Provence)

1 ounce (30 g) goat cheese, crumbled

1 tablespoon olive oil

Herbes de Provence, to taste

Salt and pepper, to taste

Place the galette in a hot oiled pan. Add the ratatouille and goat cheese. Fold down the edges of the galette and cook for 5 minutes until the goat cheese starts to melt. Add the olive oil and season with herbes de Provence, salt, and pepper before serving.

HELPFUL INGREDIENTS

Ratatouille: This dish is rich in fiber, antioxidants, vitamins, and minerals that support digestion, reduce inflammation, and protect cells.

Goat cheese: contains calcium and protein for bone and muscle health with healthy fats and essential vitamins.

Olive oil: contains monounsaturated fatty acids and antioxidants for heart wellness and reducing inflammation.

Herbes de Provence: contain antioxidants and additional nutrients that enhance the benefits of this recipe.

Spinach, feta, and tomatoes

Serves 1
Prep: 5 minutes
Cook: 5 minutes

1.76 ounces (50 g) fresh spinach
5 cherry tomatoes, cut in half
1 ounce (30 g) feta, crumbled
1 tablespoon olive oil
Salt and pepper

Place the galette in a hot oiled pan. Add the spinach, tomatoes, and crumbled feta. Fold down the edges of the galette. When the spinach is wilted and the feta has melted, add the olive oil. Season with salt and pepper and serve.

HELPFUL INGREDIENTS

- **Spinach** is rich in calcium and vitamins K and A, which means it helps maintain bone density and reduce fatigue.
- **Feta** contains calcium and protein to support bone health and is easier to digest than other cheeses.
- **Tomatoes** contain antioxidants like lycopene that help reduce inflammation and support cardiovascular health.

Smoked salmon, avocado, and dill

Serves 1
Prep: 5 minutes

1 tablespoon fromage frais made with sheep's milk
1.76 ounces (50 g) smoked salmon
Salt and pepper
½ avocado
1 tablespoon fresh dill, chopped
1 teaspoon lemon juice

Place the galette in a hot oiled pan. Add the cheese and salmon. Fold down the edges of the galette and cook for 5 minutes. Season with salt and pepper then add avocado slices, dill, and lemon juice before serving.

HELPFUL INGREDIENTS

- **Salmon** is rich in omega-3s that help reduce inflammation and improve cardiovascular health.
- **Avocado** provides healthy fats and magnesium, which are useful for maintaining bone density and reducing symptoms of depression.
- **Dill** contains antioxidants and helps with digestion.

Chickpeas, spinach, and feta

Serves 1
Prep: 10 minutes
Cook: 5 minutes

1.76 ounces (50 g) fresh spinach
1.76 ounces (50 g) cooked chickpeas
1 ounce (30 g) feta, crumbled
1 teaspoon cumin
1 tablespoon olive oil
Salt and pepper

Place the galette in a hot oiled pan. Add the spinach, chickpeas, feta, and cumin. Cook for 5 minutes until the spinach is wilted and the feta is melted. Add the olive oil and season with salt and pepper before serving.

HELPFUL INGREDIENTS

- **Chickpeas** are rich in protein and fiber, promote satiety, and regulate blood sugar levels.
- **Spinach** contains iron and calcium, both of which are important for bone health and hormone regulation.
- **Feta** is a source of calcium and protein, which means it supports bone density and muscle function.
- **Olive oil** provides monounsaturated fatty acids and antioxidants that are good for heart health.
- **Cumin:** Like all herbs and spices, cumin contains antioxidants with anti-inflammatory properties.

Fermented Foods

Many women going through menopause will experience digestive issues like bloating and constipation. Fermented foods that are rich in probiotics are strongly recommended during this time. On the other hand, if you're not used to eating them, they may cause stomach discomfort. Start small and try adding more over time: Start with 1 tablespoon every 2 days for food and 1 glass every 2 days for drinks. This can be increased over time.

Probiotics, prebiotics, symbiotics: What's the difference?

Probiotics

Probiotics are living microorganisms that beneficially affect the host when consumed in sufficient quantities. They promote diversity in the gut and enrich gut flora, all of which improves digestion and nutrient absorption. Hormonal changes can disrupt the makeup of your gut microbiome. Probiotics help correct this balance, which allows for better digestion, healthy transit, and a stronger immune system.

Prebiotics

Prebiotics are fibers in food that the body cannot digest. Instead, they nourish and stimulate the growth of good gut bacteria. Think of prebiotics as food for probiotics that maintain a healthy microbiome by ensuring probiotics' survival. Prebiotics can also help prevent constipation and improve bowel function for better overall digestive health.

Synbiotics

Synbiotics are mixtures that contain both probiotics and prebiotics. Their working together not only introduces beneficial bacteria to the gut, it also insures their growth and survival. Synbiotics offer complete digestive support by balancing the gut microbiome and improving digestion.

Probiotics
+
Prebiotics
=
Symbiotics

Probiotic-Rich Fermented Foods

Common fermented foods

Wine

Miso
(fermented soy paste)

Milk
kefir and water kefir

Beer

Sourdough

Hard cheese
(like Comté)

Pickles
(vegetables fermented in brine)

Yogurt
made with raw milk

Cider

Kimchi
(vegetables fermented with spices)

Sauerkraut

Tempeh
(fermented soy))

Lesser-known fermented foods

Kvass
(fermented drink from rye bread)

Lassi
(yogurt-based Indian drink)

Amazake
(Japanese drink made with fermented rice)

Ginger ale
(fermented drink made with ginger)

Fermented vegetables
(apart from sauerkraut and kimchi)

Boza
(fermented grain-based drink)

Kanji
(fermented Indian drink made with carrots and mustard)

Fermented birch sap

Kombucha
(fermented tea)

Mead
(fermented drink made with honey)

Jun
(fermented kombucha variant made with green tea and honey)

Natto
(fermented soy)

Rejuvelac
(fermented drink made with sprouted seeds)

Fruit-Infused Water Kefir

You can buy kefir grains online and at certain health food stores. Ask around in your area!

Makes 1 quart (1 l)
Prep: 10 minutes
Fermentation: 24 to 48 hours
Rest: 12 to 24 hours (optional)

2 tablespoons cane sugar
1 quart (1 l) filtered water
3 tablespoons kefir grains
1 dried fig
1 slice of organic lemon

RECIPE

In a glass jar that can hold at least 1.5 quarts (1.5 liters), dissolve the sugar in 1 quart (1 liter) of filtered water (mineral water works, too).

Add the kefir grains. Pierce the fig several times with a fork and add to the jar. Add the lemon slice. Cover the jar with a clean cloth or cheesecloth and secure it with a rubber band. This lets the kefir breathe without risking contamination.

Leave the jar to ferment at room temperature for 24 to 48 hours. Be sure to keep it out of direct sunlight.

Fermentation time will depend on the temperature of the room and your flavor preferences. The longer you wait, the tangier the drink will be. You'll know the kefir has finished fermenting when the dried fig is floating on the surface.

Once fermentation is complete, filter out the kefir grains, fig, and lemon with a strainer and pour the drink into a swing-top bottle that has a stopper.

If you want extra bubbles in the water kefir, close the bottle and leave at room temperature for 12 to 24 additional hours. Now you can flavor the kefir with fresh fruit and herbs.

Next, place the bottle in the refrigerator to slow down fermentation and cool the drink. When you do decide to open the bottle, be careful! Hold it over the sink and slowly let the gas out before serving.

Flavor ideas for your water kefir:

- Strawberry and basil
- Hibiscus and elderberry
- Peach
- Spirulina and mint
- Lime and tarragon
- Mango and cardamom
- Cinnamon and ginger
- Lavender and honey
- Cucumber and mint
- Lemon verbena and lemon

HOW IT HELPS YOUR BODY

Probiotics: Kefir is rich in probiotics that balance the gut microbiome. This in turn improves digestion and nutrient absorption.

Vitamin C: This drink contains vitamin C, which strengthens the immune system to fight infection and reduce inflammation.

Hydration: Kefir helps the body stay hydrated. Skin can become especially dry during menopause and hydration helps manage these symptoms.

Digestive enzymes: Kefir contains enzymes that help break down food. This makes digestion easier and reduces bloating.

Reduced inflammation: The probiotics and nutrients in kefir reduce systemic inflammation.

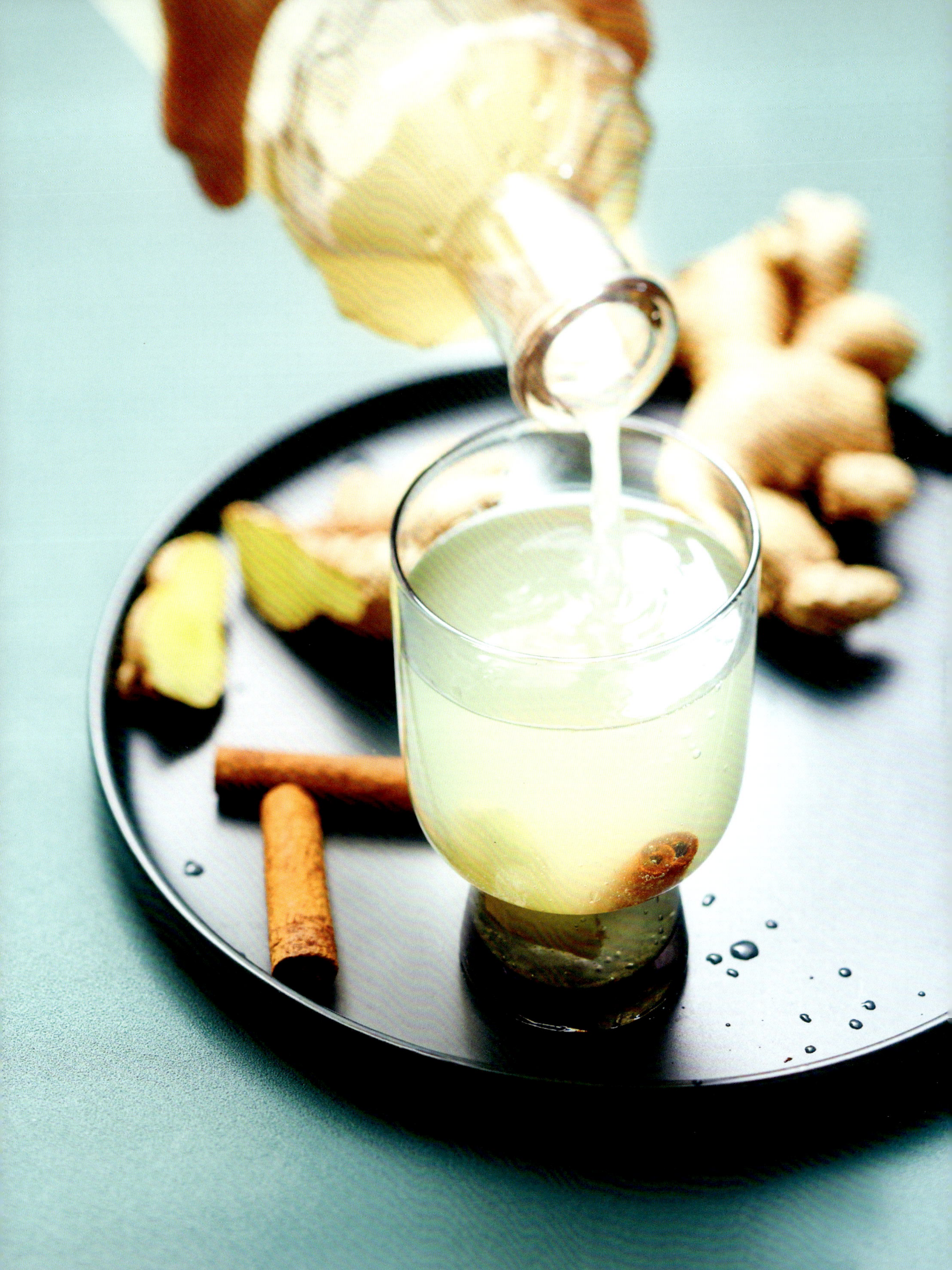

Lacto-Fermented Vegetables

Makes 2 cups (500 ml)
Prep: 20 minutes
Fermentation: 2 weeks

1 small carrot
½ kohlrabi
1 small cucumber
1 garlic clove
1 teaspoon mustard seeds
1 teaspoon coriander seeds
1 teaspoon unrefined salt
5 fluid ounces (150 ml) filtered water

RECIPE

Peel the carrot and kohlrabi then cut into matchsticks. Slice the cucumber into rounds or cut into matchsticks. Peel and thinly slice the garlic.

Transfer the vegetables to a small glass jar with a lever lid system (2 cup (500 ml) capacity). Add the mustard and coriander seeds.

To make the brine, dissolve the salt in 5 fluid ounces (150 ml) of filtered water (or enough to cover the vegetables). A typical brine ratio is 1 ounce (30 g) of unrefined salt to 1 quart (1 liter) of water, or 3 percent.

Pour the brine into the jar until the vegetables are completely submerged. If necessary, use a counterweight on top of the vegetables to keep them under the brine during the fermentation process.

Close the jar and place it in a small bowl. Air inside the jar will escape within the first 24 hours, and this will cause any excess brine to leak out. Leave the jar to ferment at room temperature (68–72°F (20–22°C)) for at least two weeks.

Once fermentation is complete, lacto-fermented vegetables can be stored for years as long as they are kept in a cool place. The longer you wait to eat them, the tangier the flavor.

HOW IT HELPS YOUR BODY

- **Probiotics:** Lacto-fermented vegetables are rich in probiotics. A well-balanced gut microbiome means better digestion and fewer digestive issues.
- **Prebiotics:** Prebiotic fiber feeds our good gut bacteria, promotes a healthy gut microbiome and improves regularity.
- **Nutrients:** Fermented vegetables retain most of their vitamins and minerals. This includes antioxidants like vitamins A and C, which support the immune system and overall well-being.
- **Improved digestion:** The enzymes produced during fermentation have gotten a head start on breaking down these vegetables before you eat them. This makes them easier to digest and reduces symptoms like bloating.
- **Anti-inflammation:** The probiotics and nutrients in lacto-fermented vegetables reduce systemic inflammation and relieve inflammation-related symptoms.

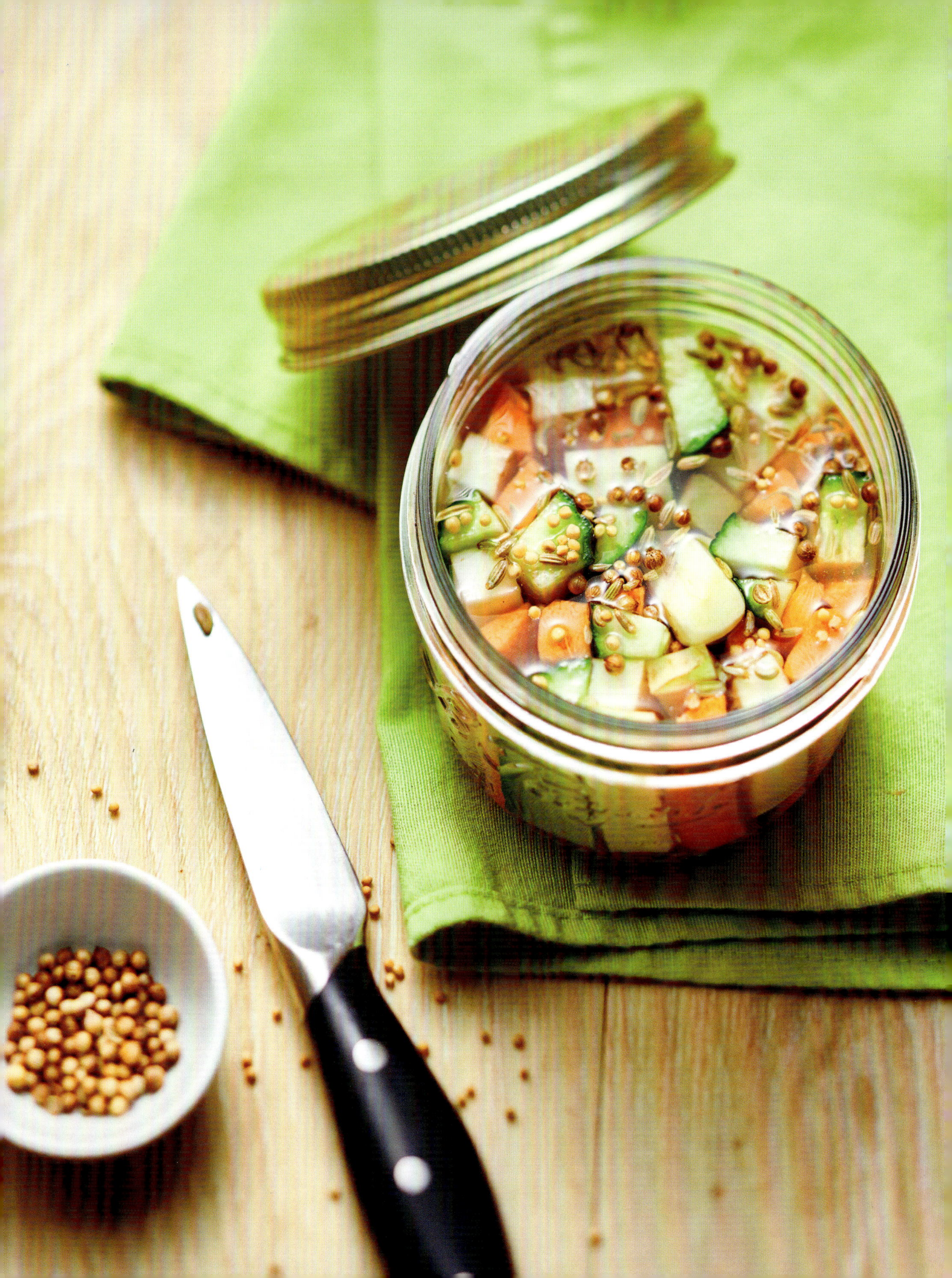

Gluten

Gluten is a protein molecule found in grains like wheat, rye, spelt, and kamut. As you may have guessed, it is also present in foods like pasta, bread, cookies, cake, semolina, and pastries made with those grains. It's a little bit like glue and is useful for binding pasta dough.

Our gluten problem today is primarily a result of the growth of the processed foods industry. Modern wheat, for example, has been artificially modified: It now contains 42 pairs of chromosomes while originally it only had 14. Several varieties have been crossed to increase crop yields and the amount of gluten in grain has increased significantly to make bread dough stickier, more elastic, and easier to bake.

Thanks to these modifications, wheat performs better for business but is much harder for actual humans to digest. Our digestive enzymes are adapted to natural wheat varieties but not to these new altered varieties.

Foods containing modern wheat are not always easy to digest, which can result in intestinal issues. Gluten behaves like glue in our digestive system and provokes inflammation because of its poor nutritional quality and high concentration in processed foods. It nourishes bad bacteria, upsets our microbiome balance (dysbiosis), and can increase intestinal permeability (leaky gut).

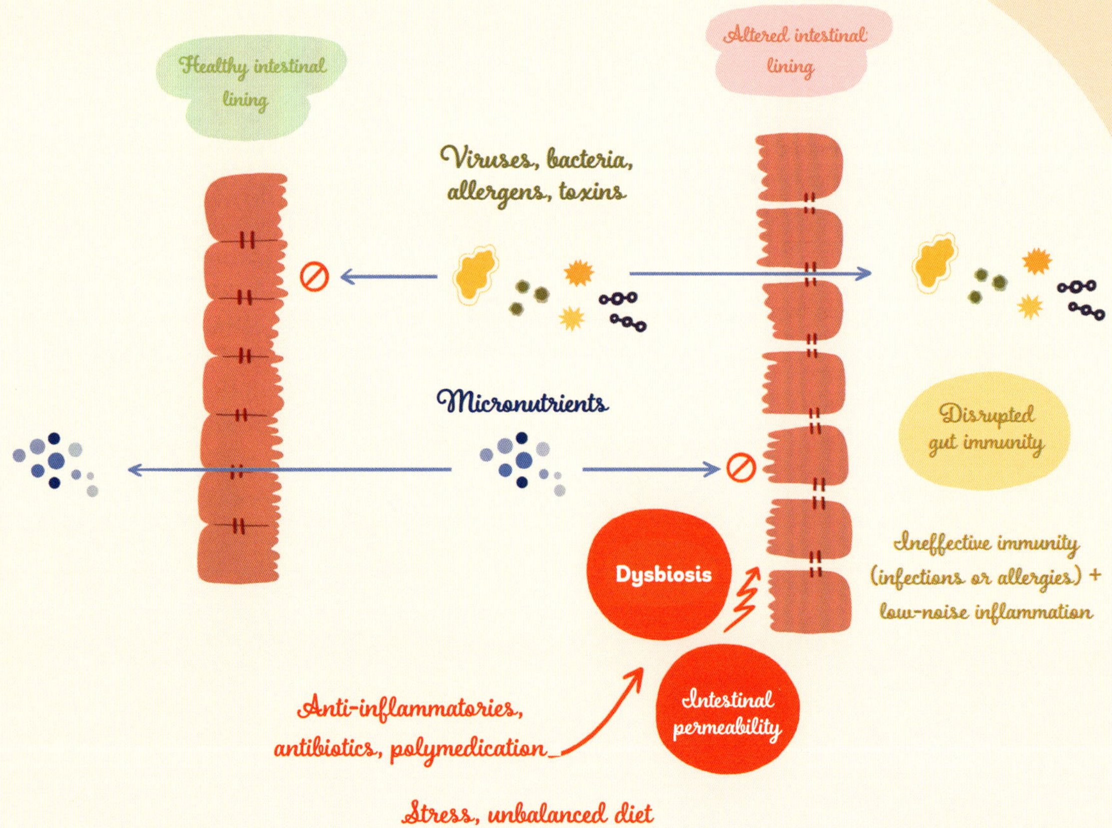

It is important to be aware that gluten is not the only thing responsible for digestive issues and chronic inflammation. Certain people cannot digest wheat properly but tolerate many other grains that contain gluten like oats, einkorn, and rye. The problem may come from other substances found in modern wheat like fructans, lectins, and enzyme or histamine inhibitors.

Unless you have celiac disease, it is not always necessary to totally and permanently remove gluten from your diet. Gluten is found everywhere, and trying to avoid it completely could become a source of stress, guilt, and even social isolation. Chronic stress can have greater consequences for your intestines than the occasional bout of indigestion after eating a piece of bread made with refined wheat flour!

A few tips for choosing what to buy

Don't fall into marketing traps
Just because something is gluten-free doesn't necessarily mean the product is healthy. Read labels carefully and choose natural, low-processed foods.

Choose sourdough bread
Artisanal sourdough has many digestive and nutritional benefits.

Eat a variety of grains
Don't limit your diet to common grains.

Stick to whole and unprocessed foods

Don't feel guilty if you eat foods that are high in gluten.
It is hard to avoid completely.

Try to cook more
Preparing your own meals means you'll know exactly what ingredients are going on your plate.

Basic gluten-free recipes

Pie Dough

5.6 ounces (160 g) whole-grain rice flour + 1.4 ounces (40 g) starch (potato, corn . . .) + 4 tablespoons olive oil + 3.5 fluid ounces (100 ml) lukewarm water. *Prebake 5–10 minutes at 350°F (180° C).*

Sweet Muffins

5.3 ounces (150 g) rice flour + 2 eggs + 3.5 fluid ounces (100 ml) plant-based milk + 4.2 ounces (120 g) almond flour + 1¼ teaspoons (5.5 g) gluten-free baking powder

Chocolate Chip Cookies

5.3 ounces (150 g) rice flour + 1.76 ounces (50 g) almond flour + 1 egg + 1.4 ounces (40 g) coconut sugar + 2 ounces (60 g) coconut oil+ dark chocolate chips + 1 teaspoon gluten-free baking powder + 1 pinch salt

Savory Muffins

5.3 ounces (150 g) rice flour + 3.5 fluid ounces (100 ml) nondairy milk + 2 eggs + 1¼ teaspoons (5.5 g) gluten-free baking powder + 1 tablespoon olive oil + finely chopped vegetables

Savory Loaf Base

4.2 ounces (120 g) rice flour + 2.8 ounces (80 g) starch + 3 eggs + 3.5 fluid ounces (100 ml plant-based milk + 2½ teaspoons (11 g) gluten-free baking powder + 1 pinch salt

Gluten-Free Savory Loaf with Spinach and Goat Cheese

Serves 4
Prep: 20 minutes
Cook: 40 minutes

1¼ ounces (350 g) spinach

4.2 ounces (120 g) brown rice flour

2.8 ounces (80 g) starch (preferably arrowroot)

2½ teaspoons (11 g) of gluten-free baking powder

3 eggs

3.5 fluid ounces (100 ml) plant-based milk

Pinch salt

5.3 ounces (150 g) goat cheese

Small green salad or a serving of fresh vegetables

RECIPE

Preheat the oven to 350°F (180°C).

Sauté the spinach in a pan over medium heat without oil or butter until the leaves are wilted. Drain well and let cool.

Combine the flour, starch, and baking powder. Add the eggs, milk, and salt. Stir well.

Cut the goat cheese into small pieces and add to the bowl along with the spinach. Gently stir everything together. Pour the mixture into a greased loaf pan (or line it with parchment paper), then bake for 40 minutes until the loaf is golden brown and a knife inserted in the center comes out clean.

Let the loaf cool slightly before removing it from the pan and slicing. Serve hot or cold with green salad or fresh vegetables.

HOW IT HELPS YOUR BODY

- **Fiber:** Brown rice flour and spinach are rich in fiber, which helps regulate digestion and prevent constipation.
- **Calcium:** Goat cheese contains calcium for bone health and preventing osteoporosis.
- **Quality protein:** Eggs and goat cheese are excellent sources of protein that help maintain muscle mass and promote satiety.
- **Vitamins and minerals:** Spinach is rich in vitamins (vitamins K, C, and folate) and minerals (iron and magnesium). These boost energy and promote blood health as well as nervous system function.
- **Gluten-free and easy to digest:** Using rice flour and arrowroot starch makes this cake easier to digest. This may help with bloating and digestive discomfort.

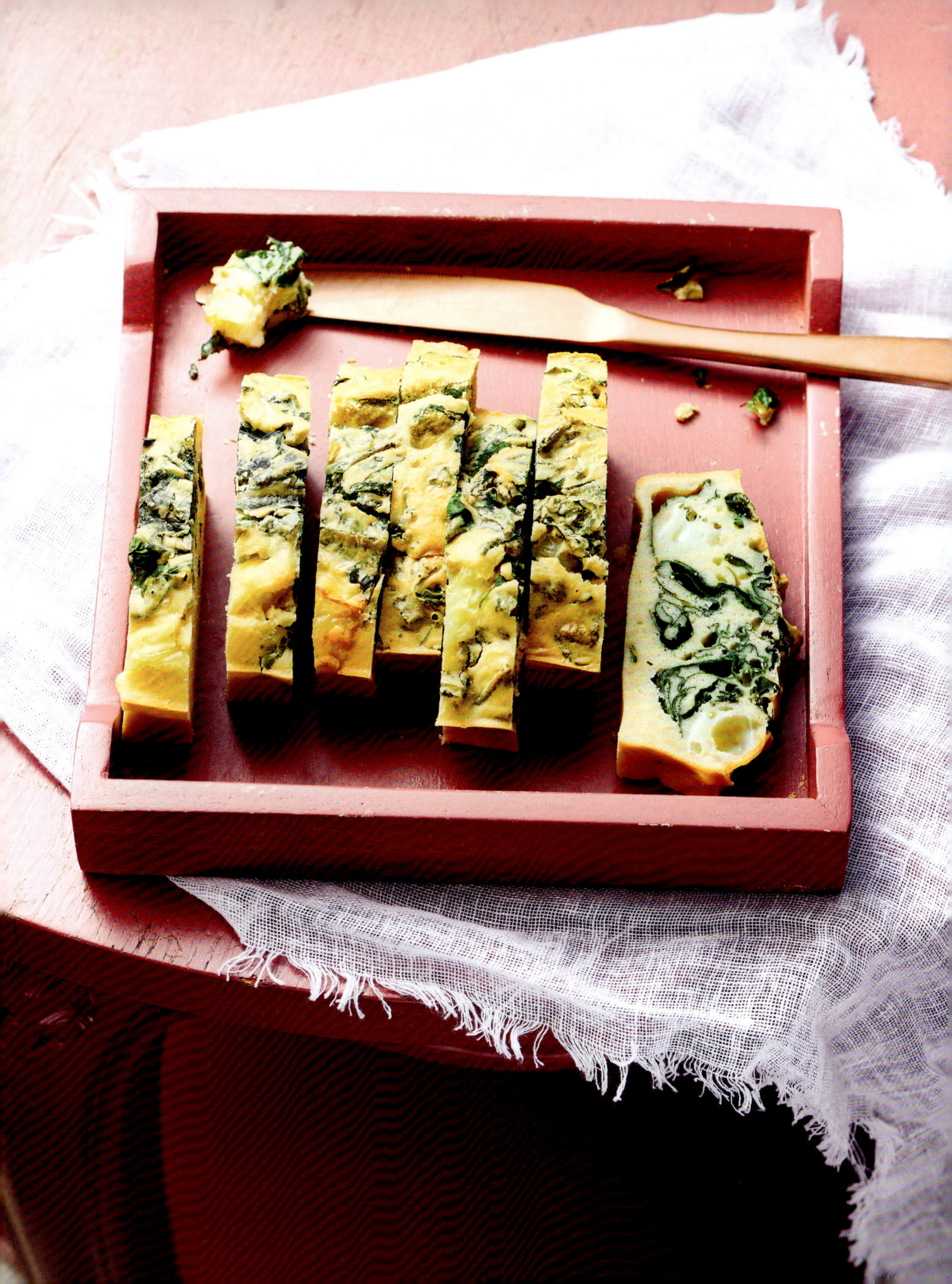

Butternut Squash Tarte Tatin

Serves 4
Prep: 25 minutes
Cook: 45 minutes

1 good-sized butternut squash

1 red onion

2 green onions

2 tablespoons olive oil

2 tablespoons coconut sugar

1 tablespoon apple cider vinegar

Salt and pepper

1 block of feta cheese

Pumpkin seeds (or sunflower, sesame)

For the tart crust:

5.6 ounces (160 g) brown rice flour

1.4 ounces (40 g) arrowroot starch (or other starch)

4 tablespoons olive oil

3.5 fluid ounces (100 ml) lukewarm water

Your choice of aromatic herbs (thyme, rosemary, herbes de Provence)

RECIPE

Combine the flour and starch. Gradually add the oil and 3.5 fluid ounces (100 ml) of lukewarm water, stirring until there are no lumps. Add the herbs. Form the dough into a ball, then cover it and let it rest while you prepare the vegetables.

Peel the squash and cut into thin slices. Peel and thinly slice the red and green onions.

Heat the oil in a pan over medium heat. Add the squash and onion to the pan and cook for around 10 minutes until slightly caramelized. Add the sugar and vinegar. Stir everything together and cook for another 5 minutes.

Preheat the oven to 350°F (180°C).

Arrange the caramelized onion and squash slices in a tart pan. Season with salt and pepper.

Roll out the dough between two sheets of parchment paper (since this dough does not contain gluten, it may crack more easily). Remove one of the sheets of parchment paper and lay the dough over the vegetables. Now you can peel off the second sheet of parchment paper.

Bake for around 30 minutes until the crust is golden-brown and crisp. Invert the tart onto a plate. Sprinkle with crumbled feta, green onions, and pumpkin seeds. Serve with a green salad.

HOW IT HELPS YOUR BODY

Fiber: Butternut squash and brown rice flour provide fiber for healthy digestion and bowel function.

Calcium: Feta cheese is an excellent source of calcium, which is essential for bone health and particularly important for preventing osteoporosis.

Antioxidants: Red and green onions are rich in antioxidants, helping reduce inflammation and protecting the body from oxidative stress.

Healthy fats: Olive oil and pumpkin seeds contain healthy fats that are good for the heart and overall wellness.

Vitamins and minerals: Butternut squash is rich in vitamins A and C and the aromatic herbs and pumpkin seeds contain essential minerals like magnesium and zinc that boost energy and support overall health.

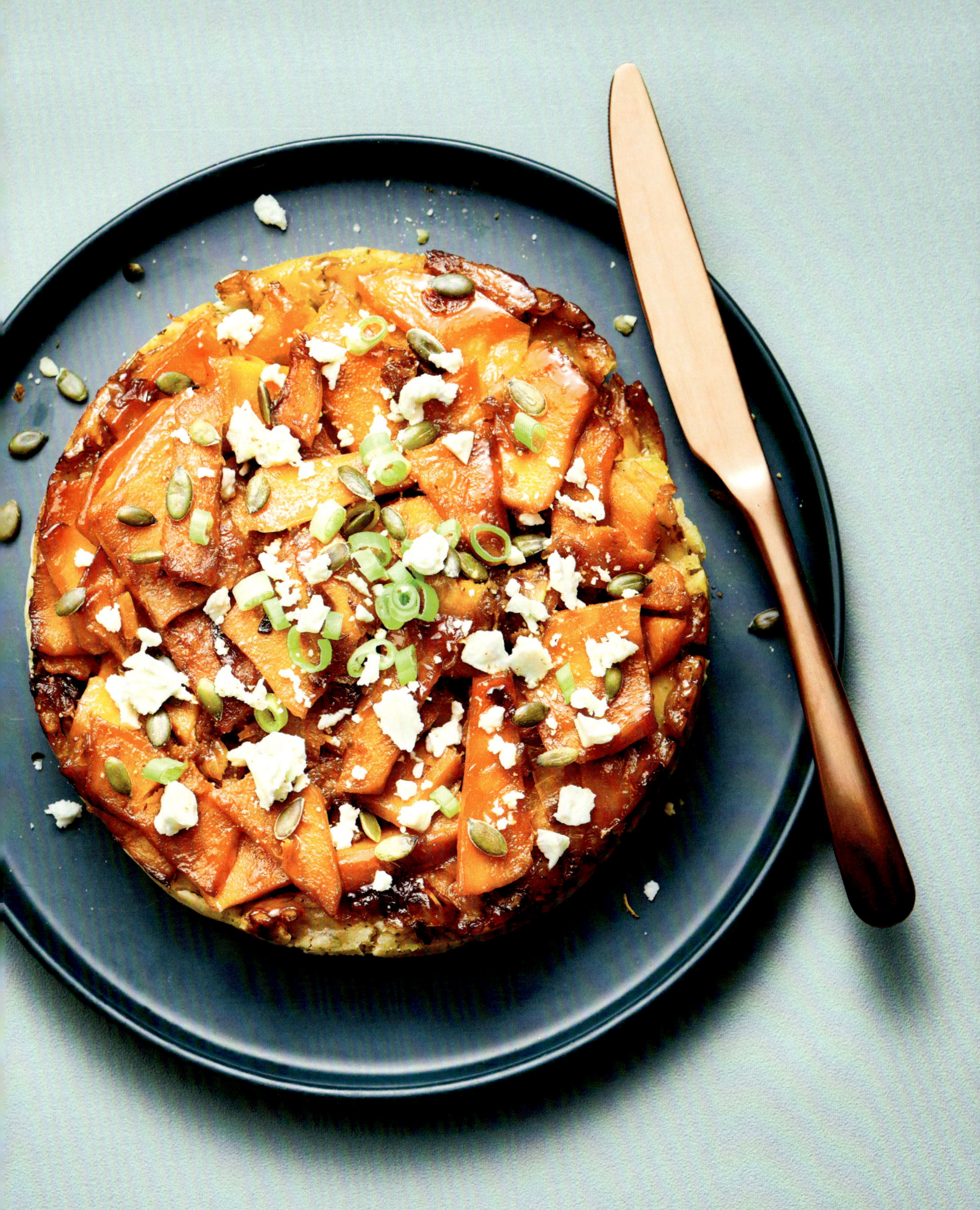

Gluten-Free Crêpes

Makes 10 to 12 crêpes
Prep: 10 minutes
Refrigeration: 30 minutes
Cook: 30 minutes

8.8 ounces (250 g) brown rice flour

Pinch salt

3 eggs

2 cups (500 ml) almond milk

Coconut oil

RECIPE

Combine the rice flour and salt in a bowl. Make a well and crack in the eggs. Start stirring everything together, gradually incorporating the eggs into the dry mixture. Add the almond milk a little at a time, continuing to stir until the batter is smooth.

Let the batter rest for 30 minutes in the refrigerator.

Grease a pan with coconut oil and heat the pan over medium heat. Pour 1 small ladleful of batter into the pan and tilt it quickly so the batter covers the entire bottom of the pan. Cook each crêpe 1 to 2 minutes on each side until golden. Repeat until you have used up the batter.

Top the crêpes with melted dark chocolate, fresh fruit, or nuts before serving.

HOW IT HELPS YOUR BODY

- **Gluten-free:** These crêpes are an ideal option for people who are sensitive to gluten and hoping to avoid bloating and other stomach issues.
- **Fiber:** Rice flour contains fiber, which helps regulate digestion and prevent constipation.
- **Easy to digest:** Rice flour is light and easy to digest, making it ideal for women in menopause who may be dealing with discomfort related to digestion.
- **Sustained energy:** This recipe offers a sustained energy boost that won't cause a spike in blood sugar levels and leave you with sudden cravings later in the day.

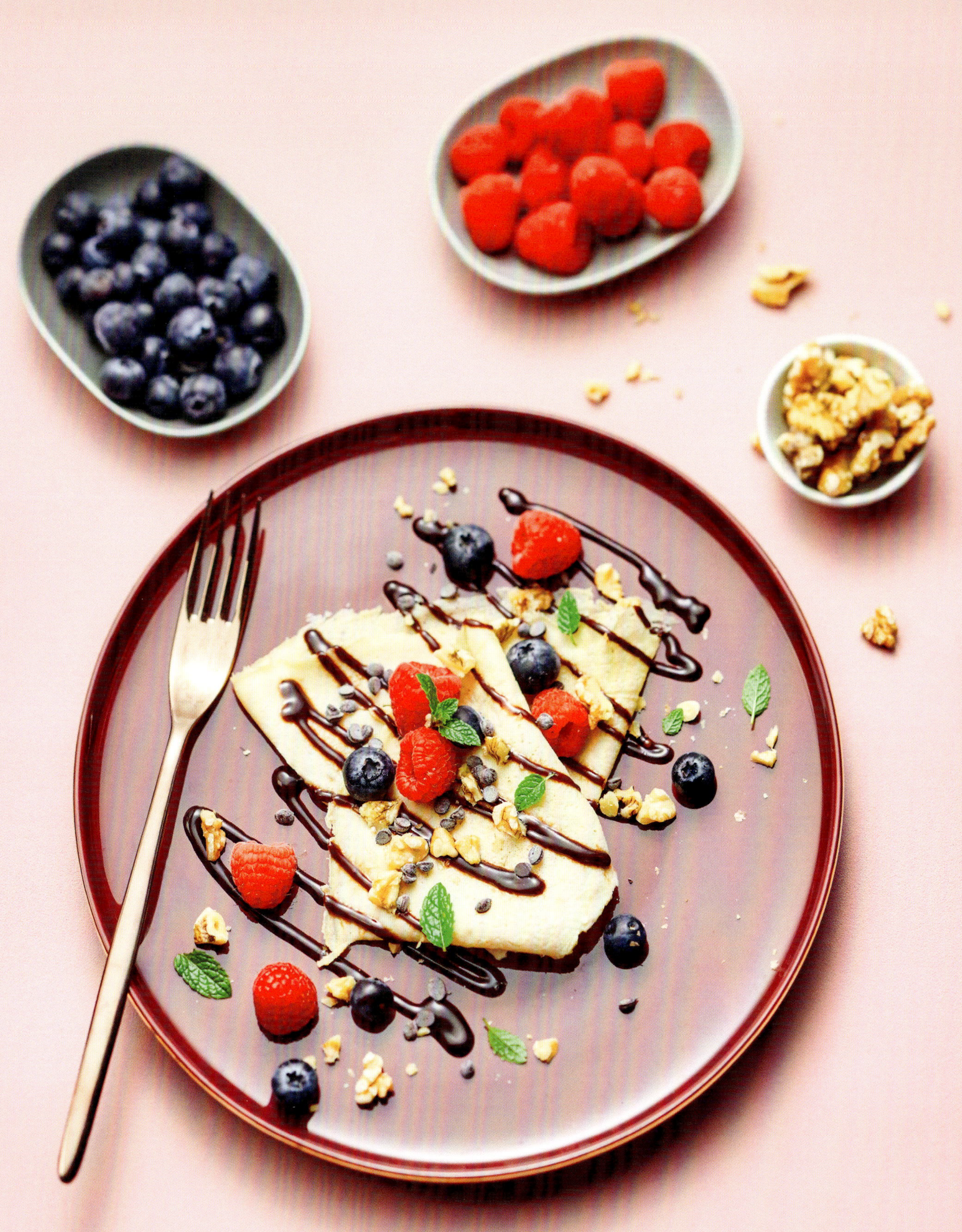

Gluten-Free Granola with Buckwheat and Chocolate

Makes 1 quart (1 l)
Prep: 15 minutes
Cook: 25 minutes
Storage: Keeps 2 weeks at room temperature

7 ounces (200 g) buckwheat flakes

5.6 ounces (160 g) buckwheat groats

4 tablespoons chia seeds

4.2 ounces (120 g) chopped hazelnuts

2 tablespoons raw cacao powder (or a cacao-maca blend)

5.6 ounces (160 g) applesauce (unsweetened)

2 tablespoons maple syrup

2.8 ounces (80 g) dark chocolate chips

RECIPE

Preheat the oven to 325° F (160°C).

Combine the buckwheat flakes, hulled buckwheat groats, chia seeds, hazelnuts, and cacao (or cacao-maca blend). Add the applesauce and maple syrup and stir well.

Line a baking sheet with parchment paper and spread the granola into an even layer ½ inch to ¾ inch thick (1 to 2 cm). Bake for 25 minutes, stirring halfway through.

When the granola has cooled completely, break it up into smaller pieces, add the chocolate chips, and toss well before transferring to an airtight container.

HOW IT HELPS YOUR BODY

- **Fiber:** Buckwheat flakes, hulled buckwheat groats, and chia seeds are rich in fiber, which helps regulate digestion and prevent constipation.
- **Protein:** Hazelnuts and chia seeds contain plant proteins that are essential for maintaining muscle mass and promoting satiety.
- **Antioxidants:** Raw cacao and dark chocolate chips are rich in antioxidants that help fight oxidative stress and protect cells from aging.
- **Omega-3 fatty acids:** Chia seeds are an excellent source of omega-3 fatty acids, which support cardiovascular health.
- **Energy and vitality:** Applesauce and maple syrup provide natural carbohydrates for a sustained release of energy that's perfect for fighting fatigue.

CLOSE-UP ON MACA

Maca is an adaptogenic plant known for its hormonal health benefits. It alleviates menopause systems like hot flashes, mood problems, and fatigue. Maca is rich in vitamins, minerals, and antioxidants that contribute to overall well-being.

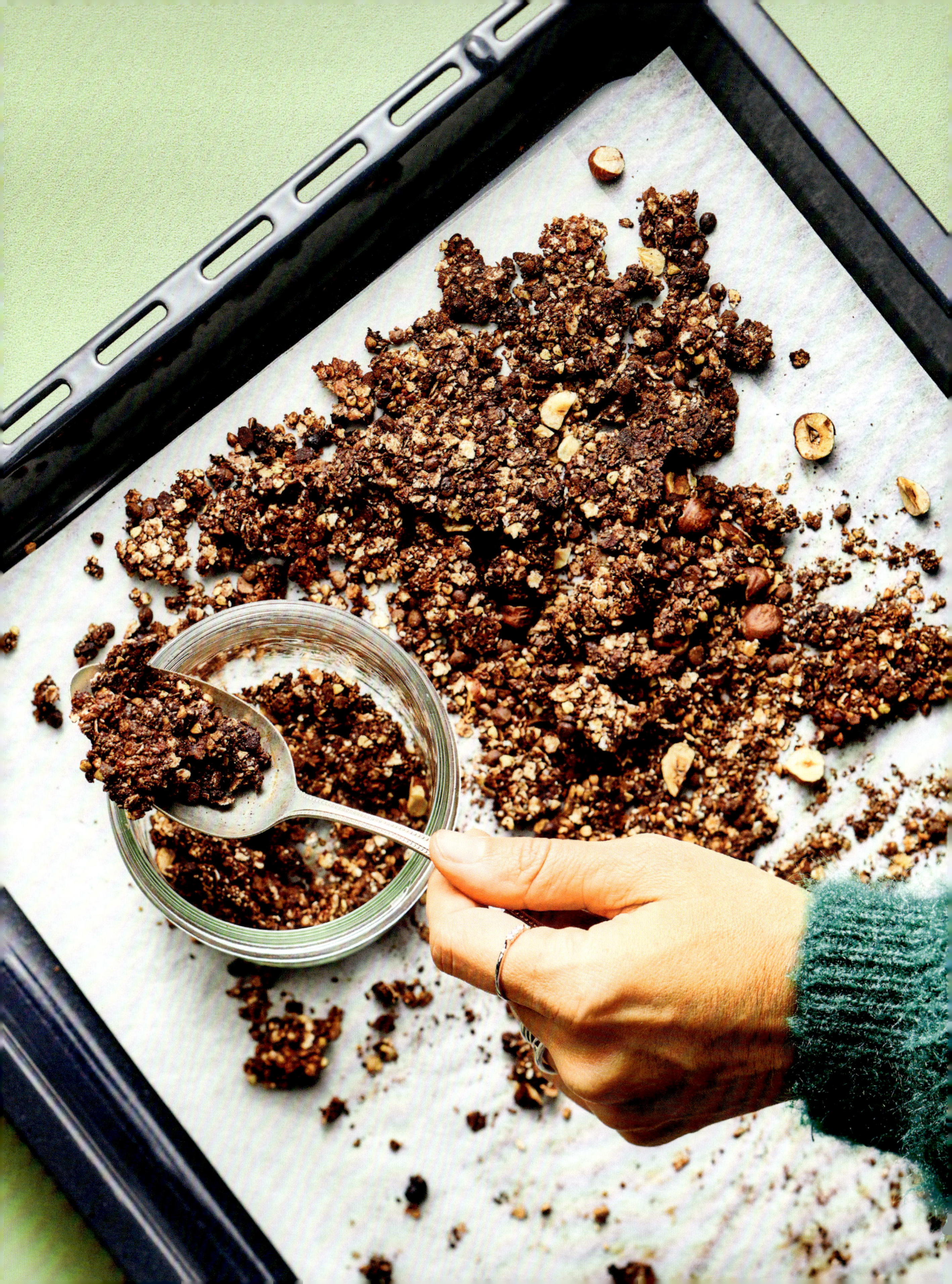

Lactose

As is the case with gluten, today's lactose problem has more to do with the processed food industry and factory farming than lactose itself.

Cows on factory farms are often given improper foods that contain high levels of pro-inflammatory omega-6s. They also receive antibiotic treatments and, occasionally, antidepressants to treat diseases and infections caused by their living conditions. These fatty acids and medications leave their residues behind in the milk and dairy products we consume (yogurt, cream, butter, cheese, etc.).

Milk is also treated (either through pasteurization or UHT processing) to extend its shelf life. Unfortunately, these processes can have a significant impact on nutritional quality. When milk is heated to high temperatures to kill pathogens, a portion of the vitamins and minerals in the milk—as well as any helpful bacteria—are also destroyed.

Your goal should not be to remove cow-based dairy products from your diet entirely. Instead, choose quality products and eat them only in moderation (2 or 3 times a week).

A few tips for choosing high-quality dairy products

1. **Opt for organic dairy products** from goats, sheep, or Jersey cows that are pasture raised and grass fed.

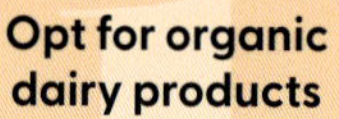

2. **Choose raw or microfiltered dairy products** so that you don't miss out on any of their micronutrients. You can look for this information on yogurt, butter, milk, cheese, and cream labels.

3. **Include fermented dairy products** (yogurt, cheese) to get good bacteria into your body and reset your gut microbiome.

4. **Eat raw butter** on toast and use ghee, a clarified butter without lactose or casein, for cooking.

5. **Vary your diet with plant-based milks:** You'll find plenty of options in organic grocery stores (drinks, creams, nondairy cheeses, yogurt, etc.).

Lactose-Free Rice Pudding

Serves 4
Prep: 10 minutes
Cook: 30 to 40 minutes

3.5 ounces (100 g) arborio rice

3 cups (750 ml) almond milk (or other plant-based milk)

1 vanilla bean

1.4 ounces (40 g) coconut sugar (or other natural sweetener)

Pinch salt

1 tablespoon cornstarch (optional)

RECIPE

Rinse the rice in cold water until the water runs clear. Pour the almond milk into a pot and add the rice. Split the vanilla bean in half and scrape out the seeds. Then, add those to the milk along with the coconut sugar and salt. Bring to a boil over medium heat then reduce the heat to low.

Cook for 30 to 40 minutes, stirring regularly, until the rice is tender and the mixture has thickened. If you prefer it on the thicker side, you can add the cornstarch dissolved in a little bit of water.

Once the pudding has reached the desired consistency, remove the pot from the heat and serve warm or cold. You can also top it with fresh fruit, nuts, or cinnamon.

HOW IT HELPS YOUR BODY

- **Nutrients:** Rice is a good source of complex carbohydrates that provides a stable source of energy. Almond milk is often enriched with calcium and helps maintain bone health. This is so important during menopause because of the increased risk of osteoporosis.
- **Low in lactose:** Using a plant-based milk without lactose reduces digestive discomfort and symptoms linked to lactose intolerance like bloating and gas.
- **Antioxidants:** Coconut sugar contains antioxidants and minerals like potassium and zinc that are beneficial for hormonal health and can help reduce inflammation.
- **Good for digestion:** Rice is easy to digest, which means it may help you avoid digestive issues.

Coconut Chocolate Cookies

Makes 10 to 20 cookies
Prep: 10 minutes
Cook: 12 to 15 minutes
Storage: 1 week in an airtight container

7 ounces (200 g) almond flour

1.76 ounces (50 g) grated coconut

2.7 fluid ounces (80 ml) coconut oil

2.7 fluid ounces (80 ml) maple syrup

2.8 ounces (80 g) dark chocolate chips

RECIPE

Preheat the oven to 350°F (180°C) and line a baking sheet with parchment paper.

Combine the flour and coconut. Melt the oil over low heat before mixing it with the flour. Add the maple syrup and stir well. Add the chocolate chips and gently combine.

Use a tablespoon to form balls of dough and arrange them on the baking sheet, leaving a little bit of space between them. With the back of the spoon or your fingers, flatten the balls slightly to form discs. Bake for 12 to 15 minutes until the cookies are golden brown around the edges. Let cool on a rack before serving.

HOW IT HELPS YOUR BODY

- **Healthy fats:** Coconut oil and almond flour contain healthy fats that are good for your heart and help balance hormones during menopause.
- **Essential nutrients:** Almond flour is rich in vitamin E, an antioxidant that protects cells from oxidative stress, and magnesium, which is important for bone health and hormone regulation.
- **Low in refined sugar:** Maple syrup is a natural sweetener that contains minerals like manganese and zinc that benefit your metabolism and immune system. This is a healthier alternative to refined sugar.
- **Fiber:** Grated coconut contains fiber which promotes healthy digestion and can reestablish a healthy bowel transit time.
- **Gradual energy release:** The healthy fats and protein in almond flour as well as the antioxidants in chocolate provide a stable source of energy that can help maintain your energy levels throughout the day and prevent mood swings.

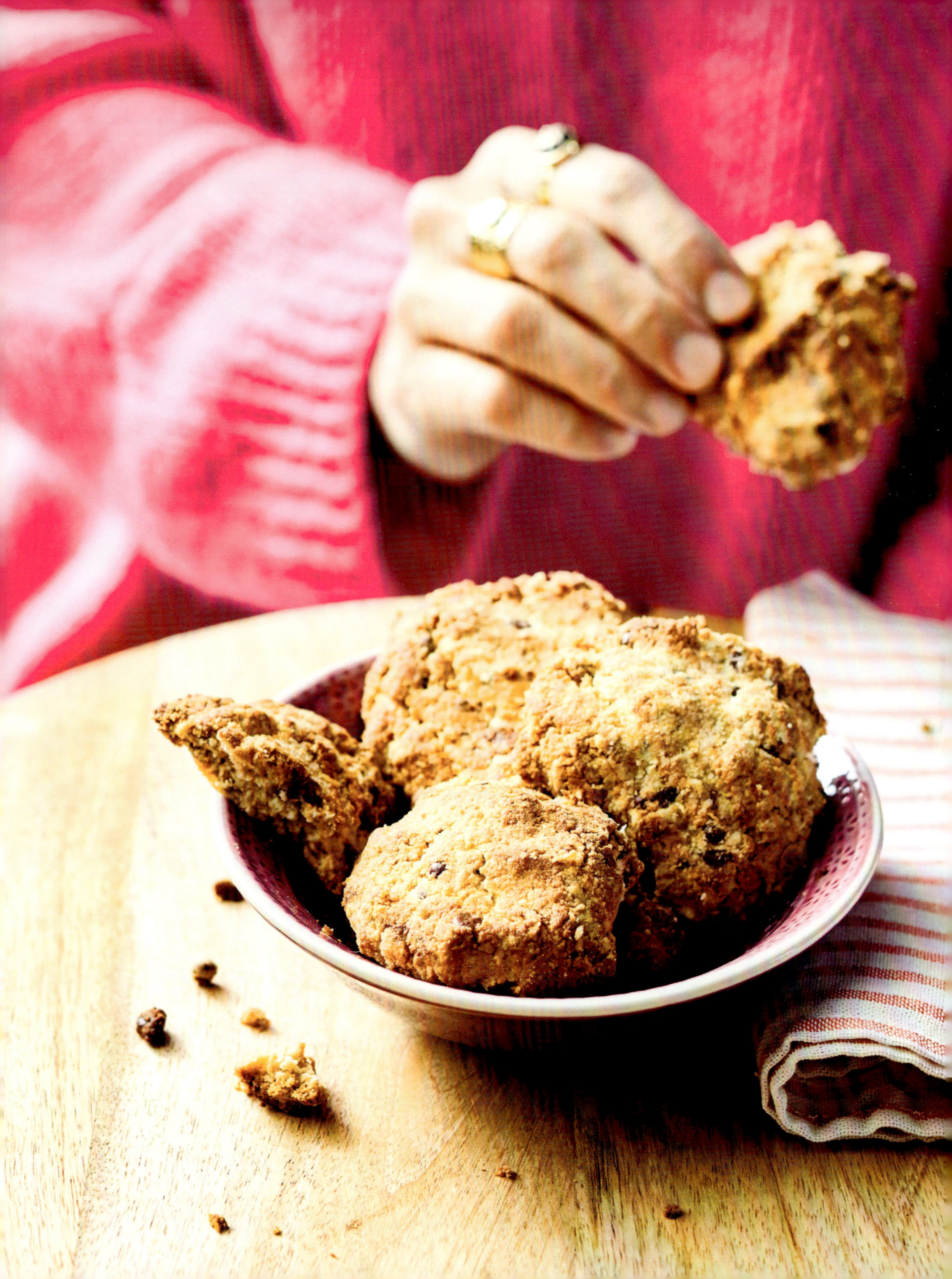

Sweet Potato Chocolate Cake

Prep: 15 minutes
Cook: 45 to 50 minutes

1 large sweet potato

3.5oz (100 g) einkorn flour (or brown rice flour for a gluten-free option)

1.76 oz (50 g) raw cacao powder

1 teaspoon baking powder (gluten-free if necessary)

Pinch salt

2 eggs

2.5 oz (70 g) maple syrup

2 fl oz (60 ml) coconut oil

2 oz (60 g) chopped nuts (Brazil nuts, walnuts, almonds, hazelnuts)

RECIPE

Preheat the oven to 350°F (180°C) and line a cake tin with parchment paper or grease with coconut oil.

Peel and chop the sweet potato. Cook in a pot of water until tender, then mash using a blender or fork.

In a separate bowl, combine the flour, cacao, baking powder, and salt.

Beat the eggs together with the maple syrup and melted coconut oil. Incorporate 8.8 ounces (250 g) of mashed sweet potato and stir to combine.

Now combine the wet and dry ingredients and stir everything together. Add the nuts. Pour the batter into the tin and smooth the top with a spatula. Bake for 25 to 30 minutes until the tip of a knife inserted into the middle of the cake comes out clean.

Let cool in the tin for 10 minutes before removing the cake and transferring it to a cooling rack. Serve when the cake has cooled completely.

HOW IT HELPS YOUR BODY

- **Vitamins and minerals:** Sweet potatoes are an excellent source of beta-carotene (vitamin A), vitamin C, and potassium. These nutrients are important for skin health and strengthening the immune system.
- **Fiber:** Sweet potato and einkorn flour contain fiber that helps regulate bowel function.
- **Antioxidants:** Raw cacao is rich in antioxidants like flavonoids that can help reduce inflammation and oxidative stress while also supporting heart health.
- **Energy balance:** Coconut oil and maple syrup contain healthy fats and natural carbohydrates that help stabilize mood and energy levels. This is particularly helpful for hormonal fluctuations.
- **Gluten alternatives:** Thanks to einkorn or rice flour, this recipe is perfect for people who are sensitive to gluten or just trying to avoid it. At the same time, this cake is an excellent source of plant protein and essential nutrients.

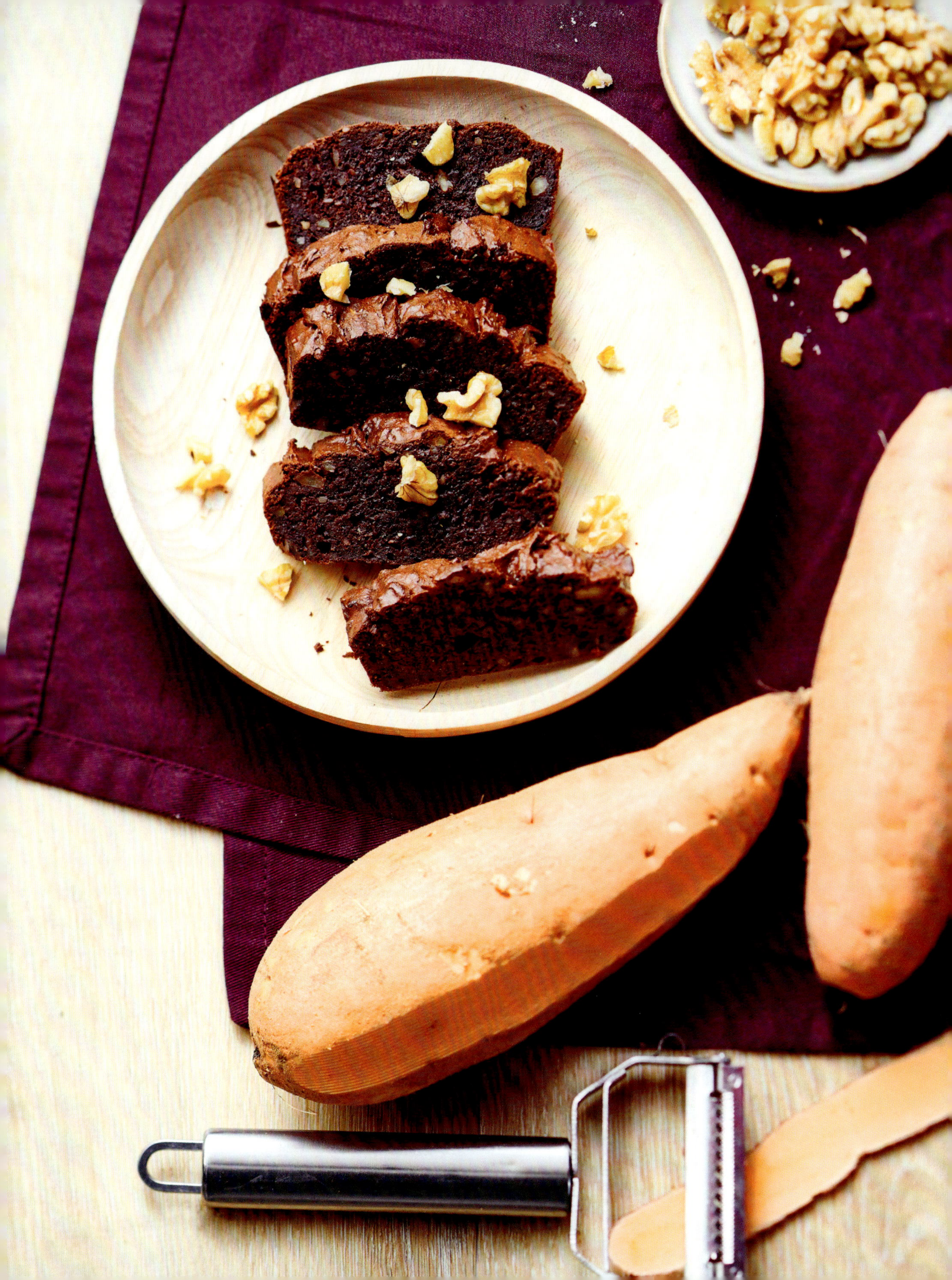

Recipes for Easing Hot Flashes and Night Sweats

Hot flashes and night sweats are common symptoms during menopause. A diet rich in hydrating fruits and vegetables can help relieve these symptoms by maintaining the body's hydration balance and providing essential nutrients.

Hydrating Fruits and Vegetables

Foods that Hydrate

Watermelon

Watermelon is 92 percent water, which makes it an excellent choice if you're trying to stay hydrated. Its high water content helps regulate body temperature and alleviates hot flashes.

Cucumber

Cucumber is also made up almost entirely of water (96 percent) and is perfect for hydrating and refreshing the body. It can be eaten in salads, smoothies, or as is.

Strawberry

Strawberries contain plenty of water (around 91 percent water content). They provide hydration and—just like other berries—they also contain antioxidants that reduce inflammation.

Zucchini

Zucchini has high water content (around 95 percent), and can be used in a variety of recipes. You may not be used to eating it raw, but grated zucchini is surprisingly delicious on its own or in a salad.

Foods that Help Regulate Body Temperature

Melon

Like watermelon, melon is rich in water and vitamins, in particular vitamin C, which supports the immune system and helps regulate body temperature.

Tomato

The tomato is a hydrating fruit with a water content of 95 percent. It is also rich in lycopene, an antioxidant that can alleviate a number of menopause symptoms.

Foods Rich in Nutrients and Antioxidants

Apple

In addition to their water content (around 86 percent) apples are a good source of fiber and antioxidants, which help regulate metabolism, improve digestion, and promote overall well-being.

Pear

Pears are hydrating (around 84 percent water) and provide vitamins and minerals that relieve menopause symptoms and improve digestive comfort.

Spinach

While less hydrating than the fruits mentioned above, spinach is rich in magnesium, an important mineral that regulates body temperature and reduces night cramps.

Foods that Refresh and Calm the Body

Pineapple

Pineapple contains around 86 percent water and is also rich in bromelain, an enzyme that reduces inflammation and improves digestion.

Kiwi

Kiwi is hydrating (around 83 percent water content) and is also an excellent source of vitamin C and fiber. These help regulate hormone levels and relieve menopause symptoms.

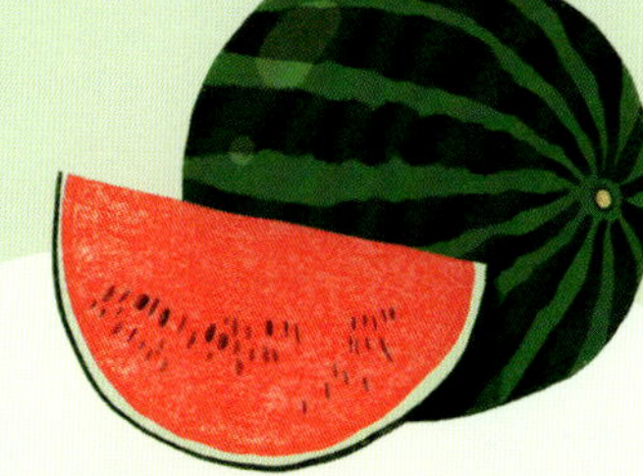

Tips for including these foods in your diet

Salads and smoothies

Add hydrating fruits and vegetables to your salads and smoothies for an extra dose of hydration.

As is

Eat fresh fruit throughout the day to stay hydrated.

Soup and juices

Make refreshing soups and homemade juices using vegetables like cucumber and zucchini for maximum hydration.

Refreshing Smoothies

Serves 1

Prep: 10 minutes

Combine all smoothie ingredients in a blender and blend until smooth.

Cucumber-Watermelon

- 10.5 ounces (300 g) watermelon, cubed
- ½ cucumber, peeled
- Handful fresh mint leaves
- 1 tablespoon fresh lemon juice

HELPFUL INGREDIENTS

Watermelon: hydrating and helps regulate body temperature.

Cucumber: provides additional hydration and quenches thirst.

Mint: helps soothe the digestive system and offers refreshing flavor.

Strawberry-Melon

- 5.3 ounces (150 g) strawberries
- 5.3 ounces (150 g) melon, cubed
- 4.4 ounces (125 g) raw Greek yogurt
- 1 teaspoon honey

HELPFUL INGREDIENTS

Melon: rich in water and vitamins and helps regulate body temperature.

Strawberries: contain antioxidants and help reduce inflammation.

Raw Greek yogurt: contains probiotics for digestive support.

Kiwi-Watermelon

- 2 kiwis, peeled
- 5.3 ounces (150 g) watermelon, cubed
- 4 fluid ounces/ ½ cup (120 ml) almond milk
- 1 teaspoon chia seeds

HELPFUL INGREDIENTS

Kiwi: regulates hormone levels and rich in vitamin C and fiber.

Watermelon: hydrates and relieves hot flashes.

Chia seeds: contain omega-3 fatty acids for good overall health.

Pineapple-Kiwi

- 5.3 ounces (150 g) pineapple, cubed
- 2 kiwis, peeled
- 4 fluid ounces/ ½ cup (120 ml) coconut milk
- 1 teaspoon fresh ginger, grated

HELPFUL INGREDIENTS

Pineapple: contains bromelain, which reduces inflammation.

Kiwi: rich in vitamin C and helps support the immune system.

Ginger: helps calm inflammation and improves digestion.

Tomato-Pear

- 5.3 ounces (150 g) cherry tomatoes
- 1 pear, seeds removed*
- 4 fluid ounces/ ½ cup (120 ml) almond milk
- 1 teaspoon fresh basil, chopped

HELPFUL INGREDIENTS

Tomato: rich in lycopene and helps relieve menopause symptoms.

Pear: supports regular bowel function thanks to hydration and fiber.

Basil: calms inflammation and improves digestion.

*Depending on your preferences, the strength of your blender, and whether or not your fruit is organic, you can also peel the pear.

Spinach-Kiwi-Apple

- 1 ounce (30 g) fresh spinach leaves
- 2 kiwis, peeled
- 1 apple, cored*
- 4 fluid ounces/ ½ cup (120 ml) almond milk (or other plant-based milk)
- 1 tablespoon chia seeds

HELPFUL INGREDIENTS

Spinach: Rich in vitamins A, C, and K, iron, and magnesium; helps maintain bone health, supports the immune system, and relieves menopause symptoms thanks to its anti-inflammatory properties.

Kiwi: This excellent source of vitamin C and fiber supports digestion and strengthens the immune system. It also helps stabilize blood sugar levels.

Apple: As a source of fiber and pectin, apples promote healthy digestion and also provide energy.

Almond milk: A lactose-free alternative that is rich in vitamin E and healthy fats.

*Depending on your preferences, the strength of your blender, and whether or not your fruit is organic, you can also peel the apple.

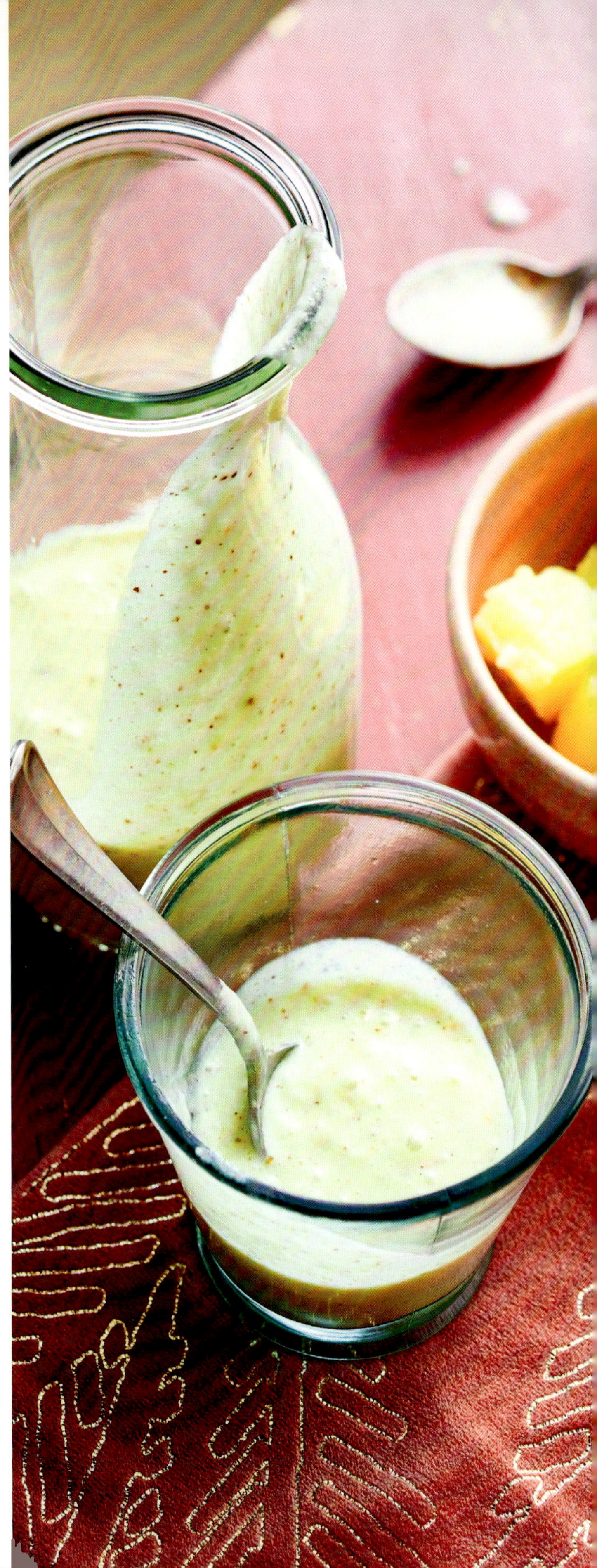

Cucumber-Mint Salad

Serves 4
Prep: 15 minutes
Refrigeration: 10 minutes

2 cucumbers
1 bunch fresh mint
5.3 ounces (150 g) feta
2 tablespoons olive oil
Juice of 1 lemon
Salt and pepper
Handful walnuts

RECIPE

Slice the cucumbers into thin rounds. Chop the mint and crumble the feta.

Combine everything in a bowl and add the oil and lemon juice. Season with salt and pepper and gently toss.

Refrigerate the salad for 10 minutes before serving to make sure it is cold. Add the walnuts just before plating for an extra crunch.

HOW IT HELPS YOUR BODY

- **Vitamin C:** The vitamin C in lemon juice strengthens the immune system and improves iron absorption. This helps reduce fatigue.
- **Refreshing:** The combination of cucumber and mint has a cooling effect on the body.
- **Omega-3 fatty acids:** These promote cognitive and cardiovascular health while contributing to overall well-being.
- **Antioxidants:** These protect cells from oxidative damage, support cardiovascular health, and reduce inflammation.
- **Fiber and hydration:** Fiber supports digestion and hydration is critical for reducing hot flashes and night sweats.

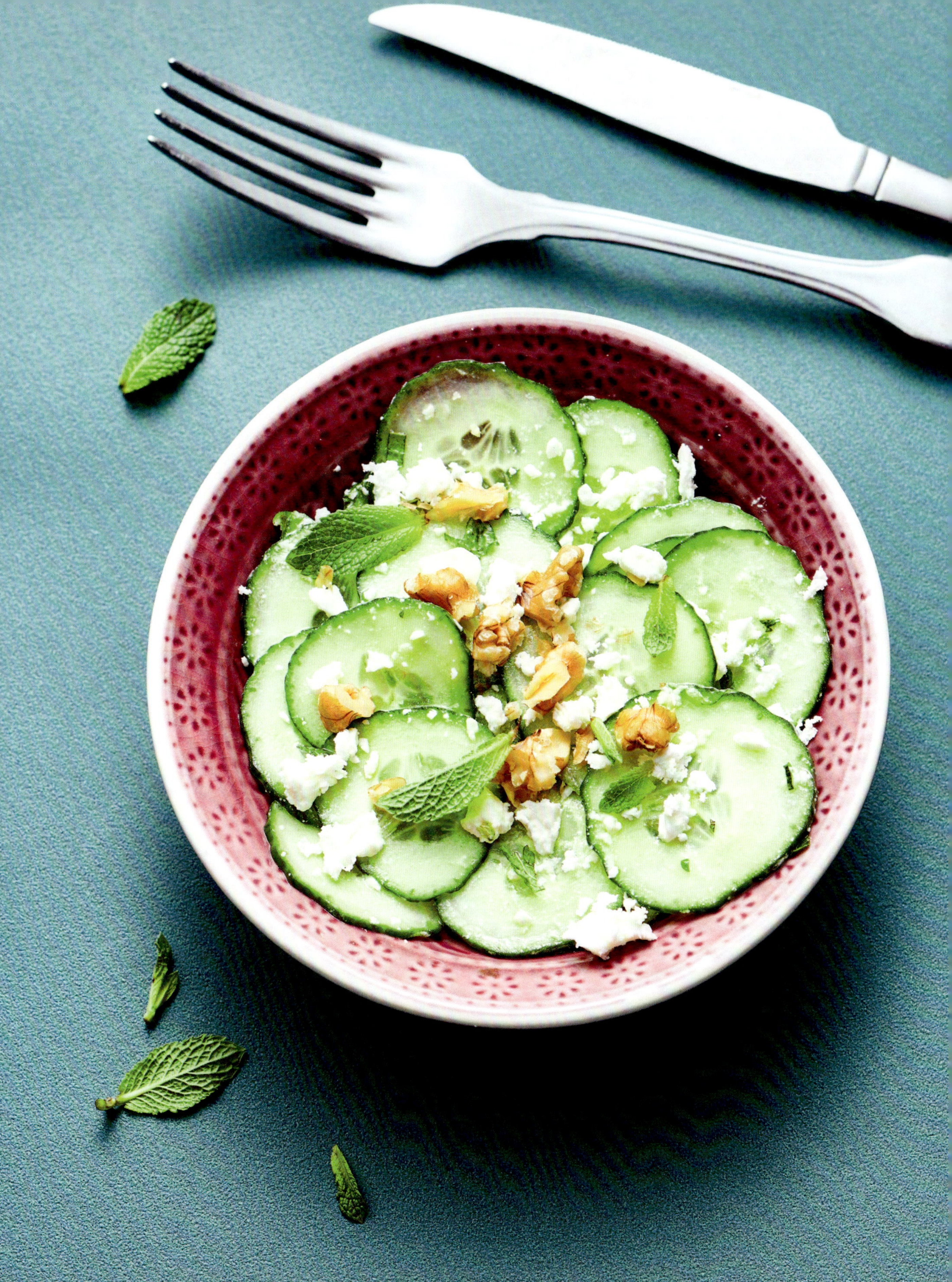

Tomato and Zucchini Carpaccio

Serves 4
Prep: 15 minutes
Refrigeration: 10 minutes

4 heirloom tomatoes (use several varieties for a range of colors and flavors)

1 large zucchini

1 bunch fresh basil

3 tablespoons olive oil

Juice of 1 lemon

Salt and pepper

1.76 ounces (50 g) pine nuts

1.76 ounces (50 g) Parmesan, grated or shaved

RECIPE

Slice the tomatoes and zucchini into thin rounds using a mandolin. Chop the basil.

Arrange the tomato and zucchini slices on a large plate, alternating colors, then sprinkle with the basil.

Combine the oil and lemon juice, season with salt and pepper, and pour over the vegetables.

Toast the pine nuts in a dry pan for a few minutes until golden. Sprinkle them over the carpaccio. Top with grated or shaved Parmesan (you can use a peeler).

Refrigerate for 10 minutes to allow the flavors to meld and serve cold.

HOW IT HELPS YOUR BODY

- **Vitamin C:** The vitamin C in tomatoes is essential for immune health and improved iron absorption. It is also useful for preventing fatigue.
- **Beta-carotene:** This vitamin A precursor is found in tomatoes and zucchini and promotes skin and eye health in addition to reducing inflammation.
- **Vitamin K:** This vitamin found in basil is important for bone health and helps reduce the risk of osteoporosis.
- **Omega-3 fatty acids:** These are found in pine nuts and promote cardiovascular health and also help reduce inflammation. This contributes to better overall health.
- **Antioxidants:** Heirloom tomatoes are rich in lycopene and help protect cells from oxidative damage while supporting cardiovascular health.
- **Omega-9 fatty acids:** These are found in olive oil and are good for heart health and reducing inflammation.
- **Fiber and hydration:** The fiber and water content in zucchini and tomatoes supports healthy digestion and relieves menopause symptoms related to hydration like hot flashes and night sweats.

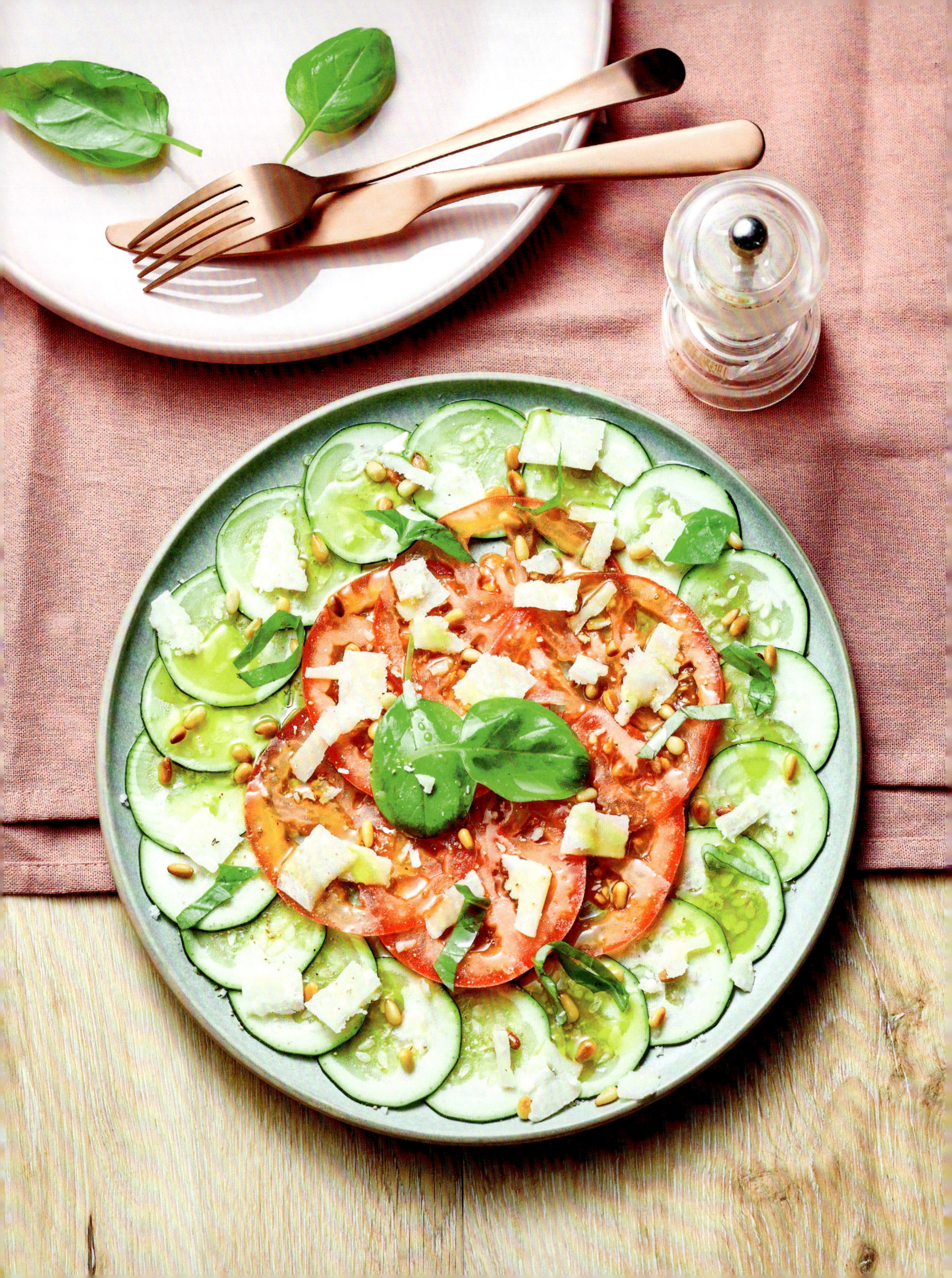

Chilled Pea Soup with Mint

Serves 4
Prep: 10 minutes
Cook: 20 minutes
Refrigeration: 1 hour

1 onion

1 garlic clove

2 leeks

17.6 ounces (500 g) peas (fresh or frozen)

2 tablespoons olive oil

1 quart (1l) vegetable broth

1 bunch fresh mint

Salt and pepper

1 tablespoon raw Greek yogurt (optional)

4 tablespoons flaxseed oil

RECIPE

Peel the onion and garlic. Thinly slice the onion, garlic, and leeks. Shell the peas if you are using fresh ones.

Heat the olive oil in a large pot and add the onion, garlic, and leeks. Cook for 5 minutes over medium heat until tender.

Add the peas and broth, bring to a boil, then lower the heat and cook for 15 minutes until the peas are cooked.

Remove the pot from the heat and add the mint leaves (save a few for decoration). Blend with an immersion blender until the soup has a smooth, velvety texture. Season with salt and pepper. If you want a little added creaminess, stir in the yogurt.

Let the soup cool, then refrigerate for at least 1 hour until chilled. Pour into bowls and decorate with mint leaves and 1 tablespoon of flaxseed oil per bowl.

HOW IT HELPS YOUR BODY

- **Vitamin C:** This is found in peas and mint and promotes immune system health while helping the body absorb iron to fight fatigue.
- **Fiber:** Leeks and peas are rich in fiber, which supports digestion, healthy bowel transit, and balanced blood sugar levels for sustained energy.
- **Healthy fats:** Flaxseed oil contains omega-3s and phytoestrogens that support hormonal balance during menopause. Healthy fats makes it easier to manage symptoms like hot flashes and reduce inflammation.
- **Antioxidants:** These are found in peas and mint and protect cells while also supporting overall health.
- **Refreshing:** This chilled soup cools the body and is the perfect meal for soothing hot flashes and night sweats.

Plants for Hot Flashes

Peppermint (*Mentha x piperita*)

Peppermint's cooling and soothing properties can reduce the feeling of intense heat brought on during a hot flash. It also helps digestion by calming stomach and intestinal spasms (this can be helpful if you are experiencing nausea, abdominal pain, or flatulence). In essential oil form, it can also be used to relieve headaches.

Brewing peppermint tea: Add 2 teaspoons of organic dried peppermint to 8 fluid ounces (250 ml) of boiling water. Cover to prevent the active plant compounds from escaping and steep for 10 minutes. Drink 1 or 2 cups per day.

Wild yam root (*Dioscorea villosa*)

Wild yam is a plant that balances hormone levels in menopausal women. It is particularly useful for reducing the intensity of hot sweats and pelvic pain. It helps the body adapt to hormonal fluctuation.

Brewing wild yam root tea: Boil 8 fluid ounces (250 ml) of water with 1 teaspoon of dried wild yam root for 5 minutes, then cover and steep for 10 minutes. Drink 1 or 2 cups per day.

Black cohosh (*Cimicifuga racemosa*)

Black cohosh is a plant with benefits from the beginning of a woman's hormonal life (puberty) to the end of it (menopause). It helps with mood problems, vaginal dryness, and hot flashes.

Brewing black cohosh tea: Boil 1 teaspoon of dried black cohosh root with 8 fluid ounces (250 ml) of water for 5 minutes, then cover and steep for 10 minutes. Drink 1 or 2 cups per day.

Cucumber Gazpacho with Bell Pepper and Fresh Mint

Serves 4
Prep: 15 minutes
Refrigeration: 1 hour

1 red bell pepper

2 large cucumbers

1 small red onion

1 bunch fresh mint

3 tablespoons olive oil

2 tablespoons apple cider vinegar

1 garlic clove

Salt and pepper

RECIPE

Remove the seeds from the pepper and cut it into chunks. Peel and chop the cucumbers. Peel the onion and cut into quarters.

Add the chunks of pepper, cucumber, onion, mint leaves (save a few for decoration), oil, vinegar, and peeled garlic to a blender. Blend until smooth. If you don't have a large blender or food processor, an immersion blender will work just fine.

Season with salt and pepper. If the gazpacho is too thick, add a little cold water until you reach the consistency you're looking for. Refrigerate for at least 1 hour so it is chilled when you serve it.

Pour the gazpacho into bowls or glasses and garnish with the rest of the mint leaves and a drizzle of olive oil. Serve immediately.

HOW IT HELPS YOUR BODY

- **Vitamin C:** This is found in peppers and mint and is essential for supporting the immune system. It also helps improve iron absorption and reduces fatigue.
- **Fiber:** Cucumbers and onions are rich in fiber, which contributes to digestive health and maintains healthy bowel transit. This reduces the risk of constipation which can be a frequent problem during menopause.
- **Antioxidants:** These are found in peppers, cucumbers, and mint and protect cells from oxidative damage as well as supporting cardiovascular health and reducing inflammation.
- **Omega-9 fatty acids:** Olive oil is rich in omega-9s, which are good for heart health and reducing inflammation.
- **Refreshing:** Cucumber and mint cool the body to relieve hot flashes and night sweats.

SERVING IDEAS

Garlic-rubbed sourdough bread: Serve this gazpacho with slices of toasted sourdough rubbed with garlic. Sourdough provides complex carbohydrates, a stable source of energy, and the digestive benefits of yeast.

Protein: Add a serving of fresh goat cheese, hard-boiled eggs, or a handful of crispy roasted chickpeas to round out this meal with a source of protein.

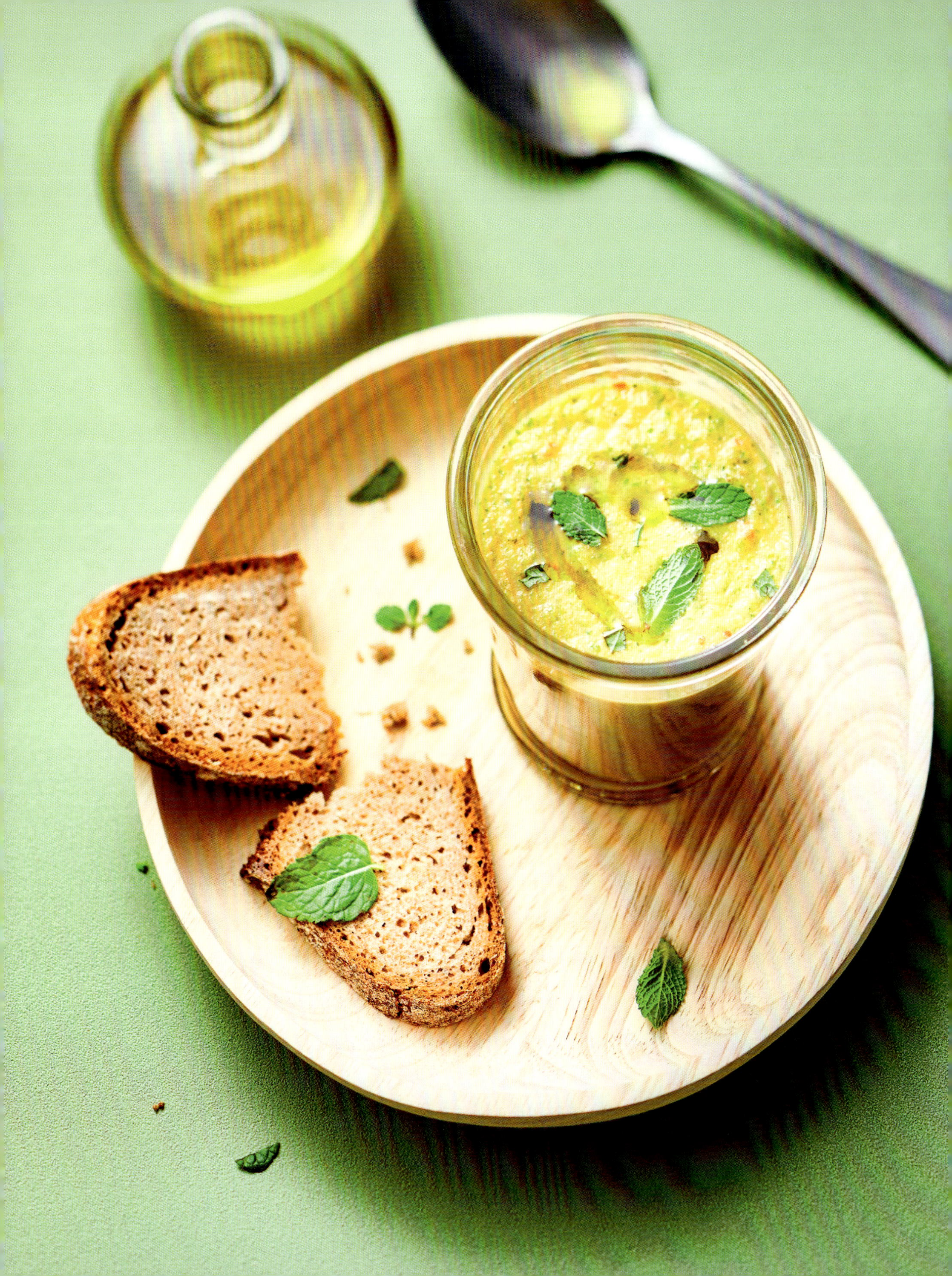

Recipes for Combating Vaginal Dryness

Vaginal dryness caused by the drop in estrogen during menopause can be a source of discomfort. Eating essential fatty acids and staying hydrated helps your body maintain natural lubrication and preserve tissue flexibility.

Omega-3s can improve lubrication naturally

Omega-3s are essential fatty acids that the body cannot produce itself. This is why you have to get them from food.

These fatty acids have anti-inflammatory and anti-thrombotic properties that can reduce the risk of cardiovascular disease.

They also contribute to heart health by reducing inflammation, improving vascular function, and regulating lipid levels in the blood.

Omega-3s can also play a role in bone health by helping reduce bone loss and promoting bone mineral density, which reduces the risk of osteoporosis.

They are also linked to better mental and emotional well-being. They help regulate mood, reduce symptoms of depression and anxiety, and improve cognitive function.

Thanks to their anti-inflammatory properties, omega-3s can help reduce inflammation everywhere in the body. During menopause, chronic inflammation may exacerbate a variety of health problems such as joint pain and hot flashes. Omega-3s alleviate these symptoms by reducing inflammation and promoting better overall well-being.

The difference between ALA and EPA-DHA omega-3s

ALA omega-3s are found in plants and are the precursors to the EPA and DHA omega-3s that are found in fish oils and fatty fish. These active forms of the fatty acid are the ones that help the body produce anti-inflammatory compounds. This transformation from ALA to EPA and DHA requires minerals like zinc and magnesium. If our body is under stress, we may be mineral-deficient. This is why it's important to consume omega-3s from animal sources.

Foods Rich in Omega-3s

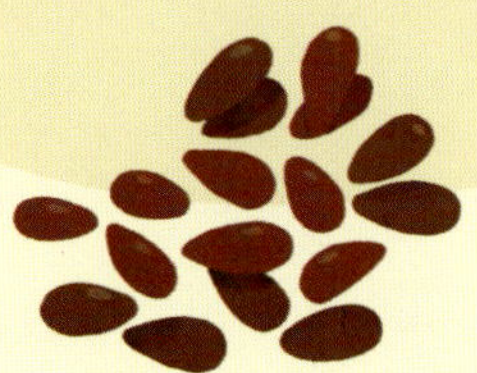

ALA Omega-3

Flaxseed and flaxseed oil
Chia seeds
Nuts
Canola oil

EPA-DHA Omega-3

Fatty fish:
sardines,
mackerel,
wild salmon,
herring,
wild tuna,
anchovies,
trout

Nordic Toast

Serves 4
Prep: 15 minutes

7 ounces (200 g) fresh salmon

1 avocado

1 cucumber

4 slices of sourdough rye bread

3.5 ounces (100 g) fresh sheep or goat's milk cheese

1 tablespoon olive oil

Juice of 1 lime

1 tablespoon capers

Fresh dill

Salt and pepper

Black sesame seeds

RECIPE

Remove the salmon skin and thinly slice the fish. Remove the avocado skin and pit and chop the avocado and cucumber. Toast the bread.

On each slice of bread, spread a thin layer of cheese. Arrange the avocado and cucumber on top, then add the salmon. Drizzle with olive oil and lime juice. Add the capers and some chopped dill. Season with salt, pepper, and a sprinkling of sesame seeds.

HOW IT HELPS YOUR BODY

- **Omega-3 fatty acids:** Fresh salmon contains omega-3s that promote hydration of the body's mucous membranes. This helps reduce vaginal dryness and also supports cardiovascular health.
- **Vitamin E:** Avocados contain vitamin E, a powerful antioxidant that protects cells and hydrates the skin and mucous membranes.
- **Protein:** Salmon and fromage frais contain protein that helps maintain muscle mass.
- **Magnesium:** Sourdough contains more magnesium than regular bread. Magnesium plays a role in muscular relaxation and can reduce symptoms of fatigue and stress.
- **Fiber:** Sourdough, avocado, and cucumber contain fiber that helps regulate bowel transit.

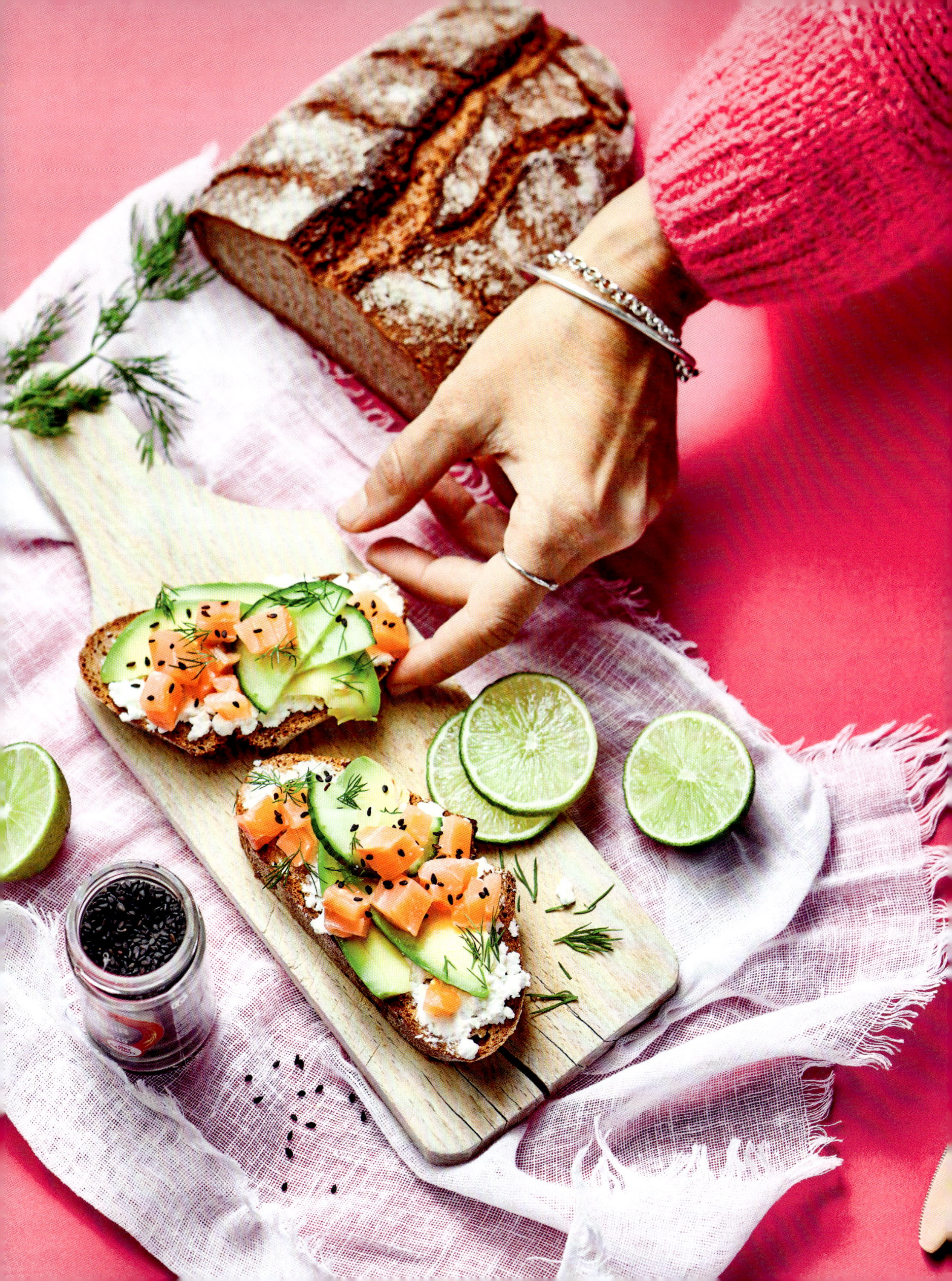

Black Olive Tapenade

Serves 4
Prep: 10 minutes

10.5 ounces (300 g) kalamata olives

2 garlic cloves

2 tablespoons capers

3 anchovy fillets

4 tablespoons olive oil

Fresh parsley, thyme, or rosemary

1 tablespoon lemon juice

1 tablespoon flaxseed (or sesame seeds)

Black pepper

RECIPE

Add the pitted olives, peeled garlic cloves, capers, and anchovies to a blender. Gently pulse to make sure all ingredients are chunky or coarsely chopped. Continue blending and gradually add the olive oil until the tapenade has a smooth but slightly grainy texture.

Stir in chopped herbs and lemon juice for a hint of freshness. Add the flaxseed or sesame seeds if desired and season with black pepper.

Serve the tapenade on sourdough toast, crackers, or as a dip for raw vegetables.

HOW IT HELPS YOUR BODY

- **Monounsaturated fatty acids:** Kalamata olives and olive oil are rich in monounsaturated fatty acids that support cardiovascular health. They also keep skin and mucous membranes hydrated, which is why these ingredients can help with vaginal dryness.
- **Omega-3 fatty acids:** Anchovies provide omega-3s, which are known for their anti-inflammatory benefits and their role in hormone regulation.
- **Fiber and antioxidants:** Olives and fresh herbs are rich in fiber and antioxidants (like vitamin E) that help fight inflammation and oxidative stress. This makes them wonderful food for the skin and mucous membranes.
- **Phytoestrogens:** Flaxseed and sesame seeds are rich in lignans, which help regulate estrogen levels and relieve certain menopause symptoms.
- **Vitamin C:** Lemon juice adds a dose of vitamin C to support the immune system and improve iron absorption.

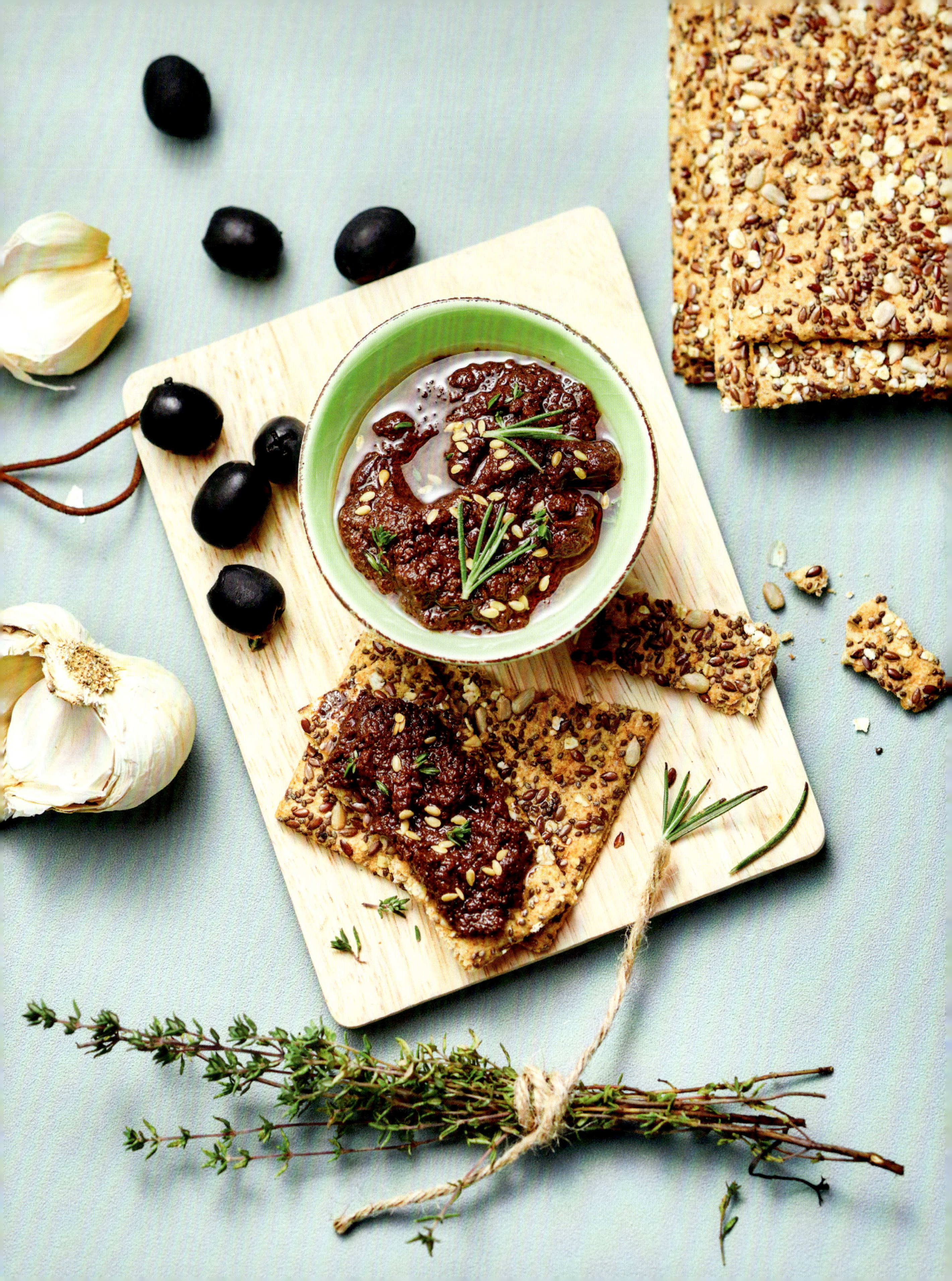

Mackerel Rillettes

Serves 4
Prep: 10 minutes
Refrigeration: 30 minutes

2 cans canned whole mackerel

5.3 ounces (150 g) fromage blanc (goat or sheep)

1 shallot

1 tablespoon lemon juice

1 tablespoon capers

Fresh chives

Pepper

RECIPE

Drain the mackerel and smash into large chunks with a fork. Add the fromage blanc and stir until the mixture is creamy.

Peel and chop the shallot. Add it to the mixture along with the lemon juice and capers and stir to combine. Cover and refrigerate for at least 30 minutes to allow the flavors to develop.

Garnish the rillettes with chopped chives. Serving with whole wheat sourdough toast or gluten-free crackers for an impromptu snack or light appetizer. To serve as a main dish, just add cooked or raw vegetables on the side.

HOW IT HELPS YOUR BODY

- **Protein and omega-3s:** Mackerel is an excellent source of high-quality protein and omega-3s, which help maintain bone and joint health and boost the body's natural lubrication.
- **Calcium and vitamin D:** Fromage blanc is rich in calcium and vitamin D, both of which are critical for bone health and hormone regulation. These nutrients also help fight bone loss.
- **Minerals:** Shallots contain minerals like potassium and manganese that are important for maintaining the body's moisture balance and supporting metabolism.
- **Antioxidants:** Lemon juice contains vitamin C, a powerful antioxidant that helps protect cells from oxidative damage and supports the immune system.

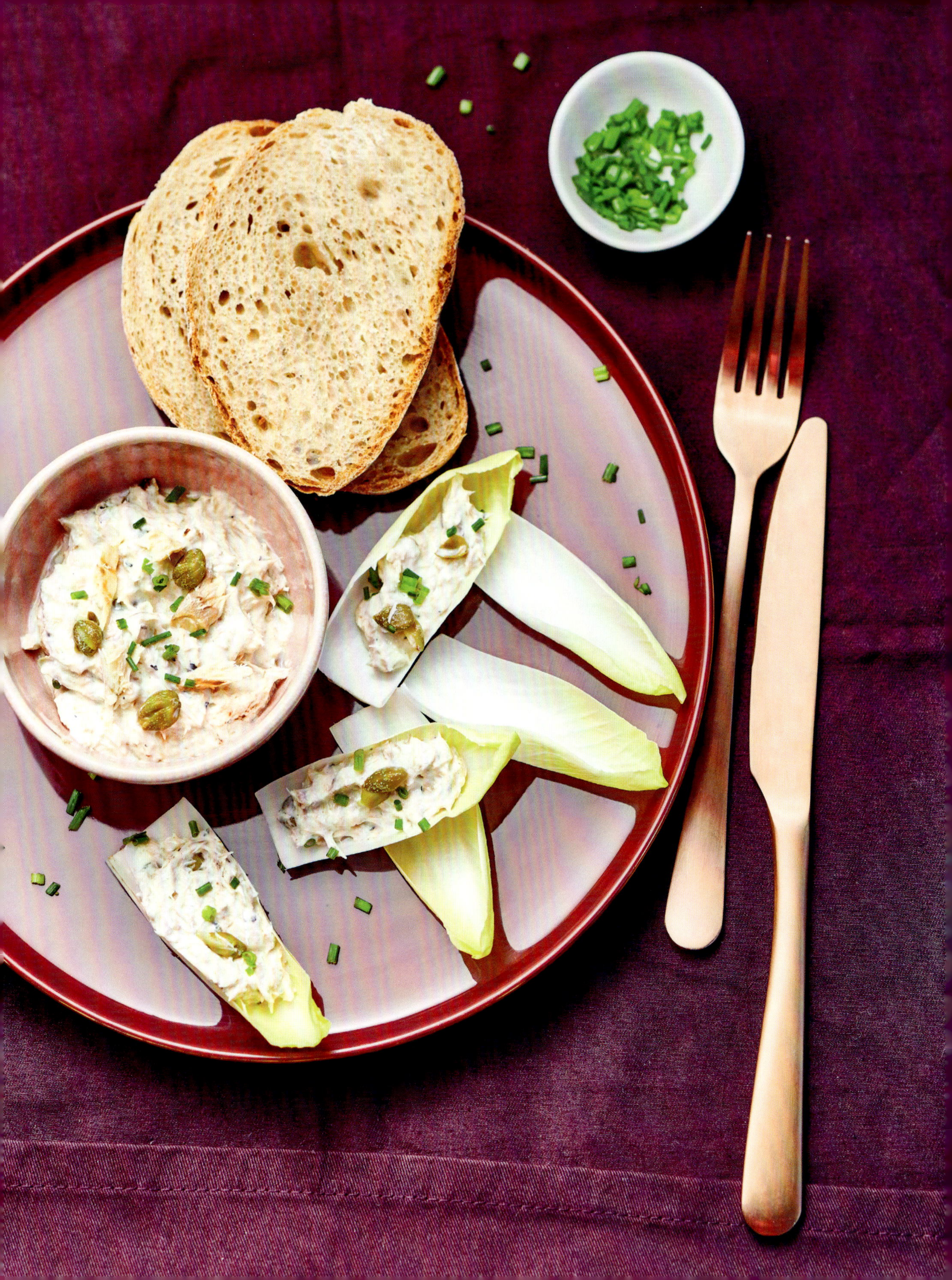

Tuna-Spinach Quiche

Serves 4
Prep: 20 minutes
Rest: 10 minutes
Cook: 35 to 40 minutes

For the crust:

7 ounces (200 g) einkorn flour

Pinch salt

4 teaspoons olive oil

7 ounces (200 g) spinach, fresh or frozen + thawed

Olive oil

3 eggs

6.75 fluid ounces (200 ml) rice milk

1 teaspoon dried thyme

1 teaspoon dried oregano

1 tablespoon flaxseed meal

Black pepper

5.3 ounces (150 g) canned tuna

1 tablespoon pumpkin seeds

RECIPE

Combine the einkorn flour and salt. Add the oil and mix using just your fingertips until the dough has a sandy texture. Gradually add between 1.7 and 2.4 fluid ounces (50 to 70 ml) of lukewarm water until you are able to form a ball. Knead a few times and cover with a kitchen towel before letting the dough rest for 10 minutes in the refrigerator.

Preheat the oven to 350°F (180°C).

Roll out the dough between 2 sheets of parchment paper and transfer to a tart pan. Prick the bottom of the tart with a fork and prebake for 5 minutes.

Sauté the spinach in a pan with a little olive oil until wilted. Drain well.

Beat the eggs together with the milk. Add the herbs, flaxseed meal, and season with pepper. Drain the tuna and crumble it into the egg mixture. Now add the spinach.

Pour the filling into the prebaked crust. Sprinkle with pumpkin seeds for an added crunch and extra nutrients then bake for 30 to 35 minutes until the quiche is golden and firm. Serve with a green salad.

HOW IT HELPS YOUR BODY

- **Protein:** Tuna is an excellent source of protein and omega-3s, which help reduce inflammation and support cardiovascular health. The eggs in this recipe also provide protein.
- **Fiber and antioxidants:** Spinach is rich in fiber, antioxidants, and vitamin K, which is good for bone health. Its magnesium content also helps reduce stress and anxiety.
- **Healthy fats:** Olive oil and flaxseed are rich in omega-3s. These fatty acids are essential for hydrating the body's mucous membranes (including those found in the vagina) and supporting hormonal balance during menopause.
- **Magnesium and zinc:** Pumpkin seeds are rich in magnesium, which supports the nervous system and helps manage stress-related symptoms. They also contain zinc, which plays an important role in hormone regulation.
- **Vitamin E:** Vitamin E is a powerful antioxidant found in olive oil that protects cells and maintains mucous membrane elasticity. This is what makes it such a helpful ally against vaginal dryness.

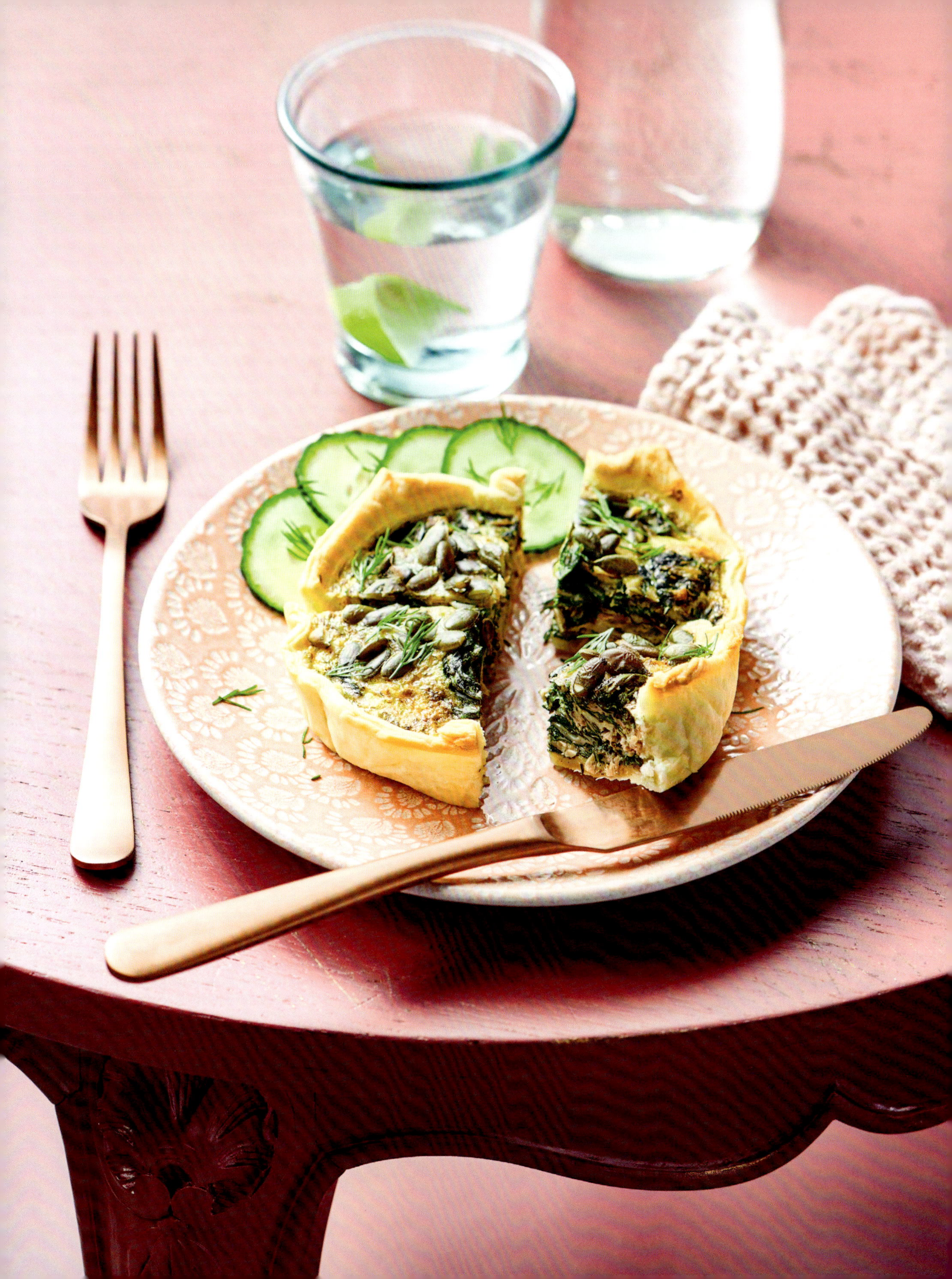

Sea Bream Ceviche Bowl

Serves 4
Prep: 20 minutes
Marinate: 10 minutes
Cook: 15 minutes

200 g brown basmati rice

1 mango

1 avocado

200 g fresh sea bream

1 pomegranate

Handful fresh cilantro

2 tablespoons tamari (or gluten-free soy sauce)

Juice of 1 lime

2 tablespoons pumpkin seeds

1 tablespoon sesame seeds

1 tablespoon sesame oil

1 small red chili pepper (optional)

RECIPE

Rinse the rice under cold water and cook in a pot following the instructions on the packet. Drain the rice and let cool.

Remove the skin from the mango and avocado. Cut the mango, avocado, and sea bream into cubes. Remove the pomegranate seeds. Chop the cilantro.

Season the fish with the tamari and lime juice. Marinate for at least 10 minutes.

Divide the rice into 4 bowls. Top with the sea bream, mango, avocado, and pomegranate seeds. Sprinkle over the pumpkin and sesame seeds. Drizzle with sesame oil. If you want, you can add a few slices of chopped chili pepper. Garnish with chopped cilantro and serve immediately.

HOW IT HELPS YOUR BODY

- **Protein and omega-3s:** Sea bream is an excellent source of lean protein and omega-3s, both of which are essential for bone health and hormone regulation. Omega-3s help reduce inflammation and alleviate vaginal dryness.
- **Fiber and vitamins:** Mango and avocado provide fiber and essential vitamins A and E. Pomegranate is high in antioxidants and vitamin C, which helps fight against oxidative stress and keeps skin healthy.
- **Minerals and healthy fats:** Pumpkin seeds are rich in zinc, an important mineral for hormonal health. Sesame oil contains healthy fats and lignans that can help balance hormone levels.
- **Improved bowel function:** Brown basmati rice contains fiber, which promotes regular bowel function and healthy digestion.

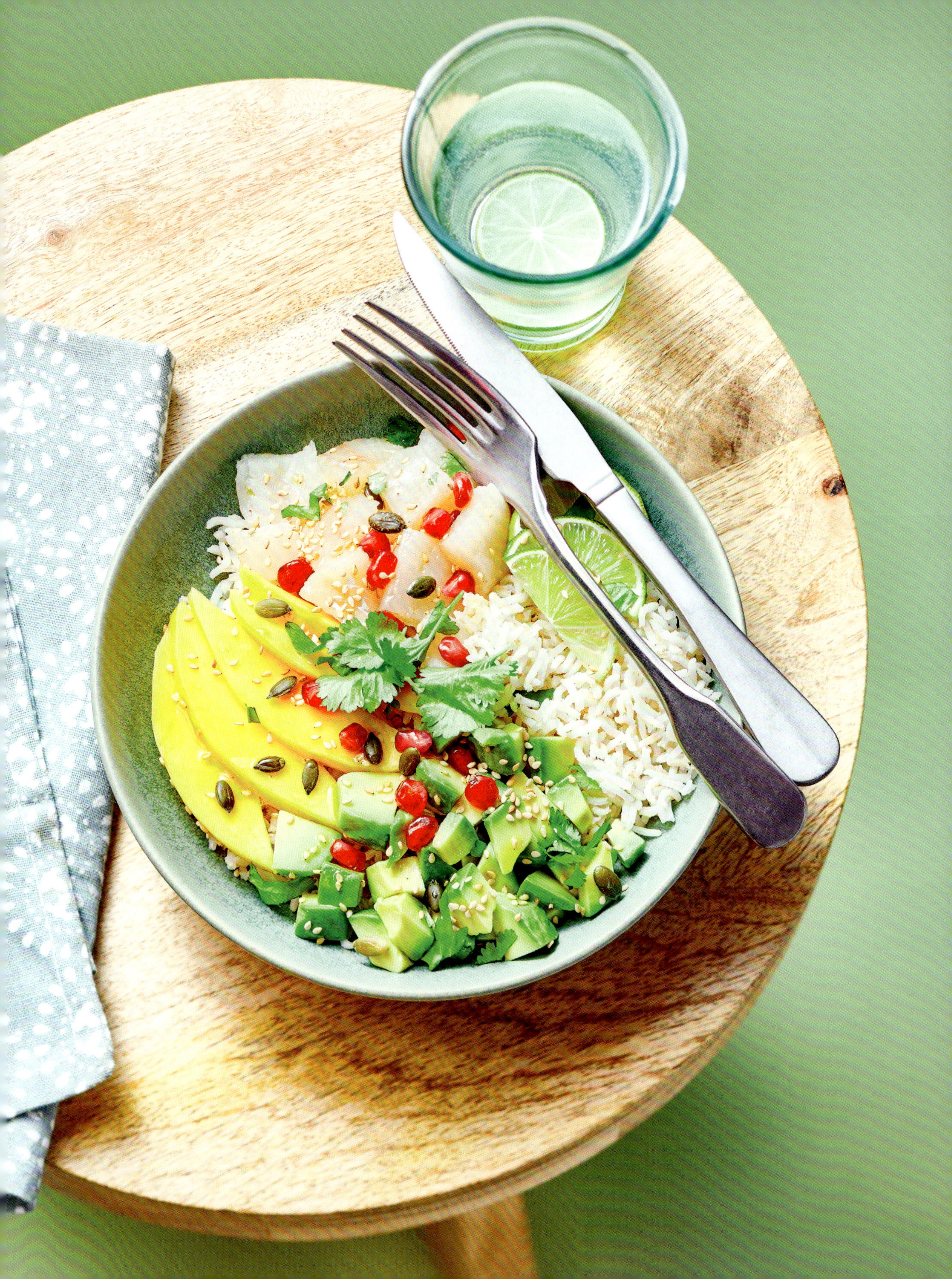

Recipes for Cardiovascular Health

Declining hormone levels during menopause may increase your risk of heart problems. A diet with plenty of high-quality fatty acids and the right balance of omega-3s and omega-6s will give your cardiovascular system a much-needed boost.

Saturated and Unsaturated Fats

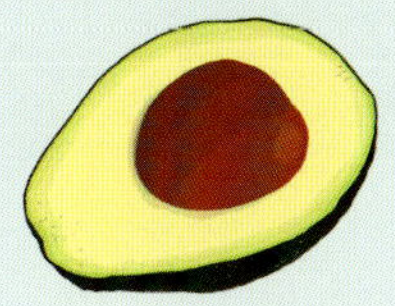

Saturated fats

Saturated fats are usually of animal origin. They are found in foods like red meat, deli meat, butter, cheese, and cream, as well as certain plant oils like coconut oil and palm oil. Their unique chemical structure—there are no double bonds between their carbon atoms—means that saturated fats are solid at room temperature.

Overconsumption of saturated fats is associated with an increase in LDL cholesterol levels. This kind of cholesterol can accumulate in artery walls and form plaques, which are a major risk factor for cardiovascular disease. Keep in mind, though, that it is only an overconsumption of these saturated fats that causes problems. There are plenty of other benefits to eating meat, raw dairy products, and plant oils.

Unsaturated fats

Unsaturated fats come primarily from plants and are liquid at room temperature. These fats have one or more double bonds between their carbon atoms and this impacts their shape and the way they behave in the body.

MUFA fats: monounsaturated fatty acids (omega-9)

Monounsaturated fatty acids are known for their ability to reduce LDL cholesterol while boosting HDL cholesterol levels. HDL acts as a cholesterol transporter and sends LDL from the arteries to the liver where it can be broken down and eliminated from the body.

Food sources: nuts, olive oil, avocado (and avocado oil), canola oil . . .

PUFA fats: polyunsaturated fatty acids (omega-3 and omega-6)

Omega-3s and omega-6s are essential fatty acids: the body cannot produce them and we can only get them from the food we eat.

Omega-3s (found in fatty fish like salmon, sardines, mackerel, flaxseed, chia seed, and nuts) are known for their anti-inflammatory properties. They help reduce blood triglyceride levels, improve endothelial function (this is our blood vessels' ability to dilate and contract), and reduce the risk of blood clots. Many studies have also indicated that omega-3s can lower the risk of death by heart disease.

Omega-6s (found in plant oils like sunflower oil, corn oil, and soybean oil) also play an important role in regulating cardiovascular and immune function. However, a diet that is too high in omega-6s without enough omega-3s can promote inflammation. This is why it is critical to maintain a good balance between these two kinds of polyunsaturated fatty acids. When in doubt, make a diet rich in omega-3s your priority.

The right omega-3 to omega-6 ratio

It is important to maintain a balance between the amount of omega-3 and omega-6 in your diet. This balance plays a crucial role in the body's health because it has a direct influence on its ability to regulate inflammation. Official recommendations suggest that an ideal ratio of omega-6s to omega-3s is 5:1. Unfortunately, thanks to our increased consumption of processed foods containing sunflower oil and the use of intensive farming practices where animals are primarily fed foods that are rich in omega-6 (like soy and corn), in many places this ratio has drifted significantly off course. In France, for instance, the ratio is 18:1. Consuming an excess of omega-6s —and creating a fatty acid imbalance in the body—is the root cause of multiple inflammatory conditions and can make a variety of health problems even worse.

5 Sauce Ideas

Tahini-Yogurt Sauce

• 2 tablespoons tahini • 3 tablespoons yogurt made with goat or sheep's milk • 1 tablespoon lemon juice • 1 tablespoon olive oil • 1 crushed garlic clove • Salt and pepper, to taste

Pour the ingredients into a bowl and whisk together to combine.

Avocado and Apple Cider Vinaigrette

½ avocado, blended or crushed • 2 tablespoons raw apple cider vinegar • 3 tablespoons walnut or olive oil • 1 teaspoon Dijon mustard • Salt and pepper, to taste

Pour the ingredients into a bowl and whisk together to combine.

Flaxseed Oil and Lemon Vinaigrette

3 tablespoons flaxseed oil • Juice of ½ lemon • 1 tablespoon raw apple cider vinegar • 1 teaspoon mustard • Salt and pepper, to taste

Pour the ingredients into a bowl and whisk together to combine.

Creamy Sesame Oil and Ginger Sauce

2 tablespoons sesame oil • 3 tablespoons plain yogurt (goat or sheep's milk) • 1 tablespoon rice vinegar • 1 tablespoon tamari • 1 tablespoon fresh ginger, grated • 1 teaspoon honey • Salt and pepper, to taste

Pour the ingredients into a bowl and whisk together to combine.

Hemp Oil and Cilantro Sauce

½ bunch cilantro, chopped • 3 tablespoons hemp oil • Juice of ½ lemon • 1 tablespoon balsamic vinegar • 1 crushed garlic clove • Salt and pepper, to taste

If you have one, use a mortar and pestle to grind the cilantro and oil together. Add the rest of the ingredients and whisk together to combine.

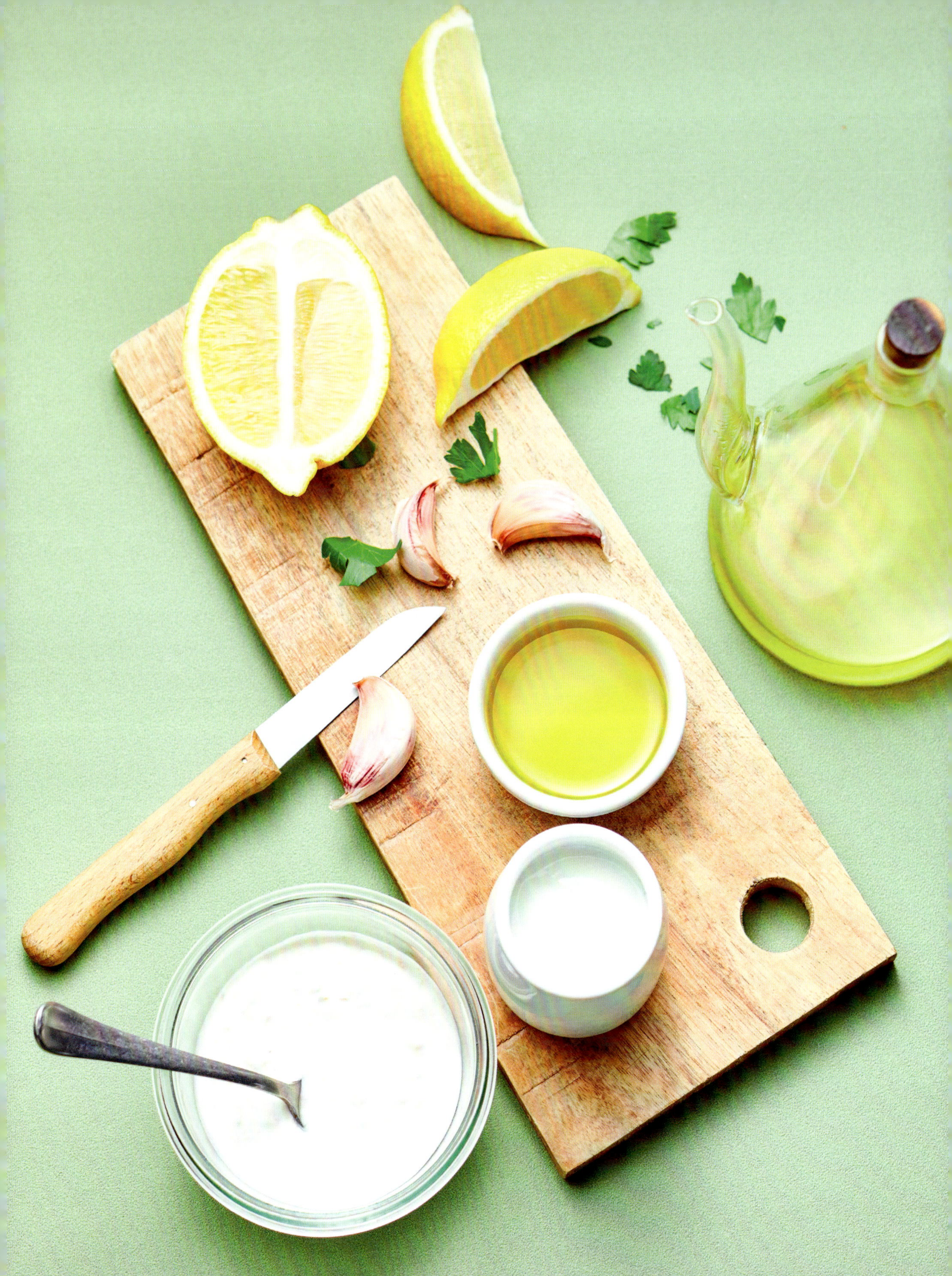

Bright Vegetable Salad with Lentils and Avocado

Serves 4
Prep: 20 minutes

2 carrots

1 red bell pepper

1 yellow bell pepper

1 avocado

1 cucumber

1 red onion

1 bunch fresh cilantro or parsley

14 ounces (400 g) lentils, cooked or canned

Arugula or lamb's lettuce

3 tablespoons olive oil

Juice of 1 lemon

1 tablespoon apple cider vinegar

1 tablespoon flaxseed or chia seeds

Feta crumbles

Salt and pepper, to taste

RECIPE

Peel the carrots and cut into matchsticks or slice into thin rounds. Cut the peppers, avocado, and cucumber into cubes. Peel and thinly slice the onion. Chop the herbs. Drain and rinse the lentils (cook them yourself if you can).

Combine the lentils with the carrots, peppers, cucumber, onion, herbs, and arugula.

In a separate bowl, combine the oil, lemon juice, vinegar, and flaxseed or chia seeds. Season with salt and pepper and pour the vinaigrette over the salad. Toss gently to coat the vegetables. Top with avocado pieces just before serving to keep them from oxidizing. Sprinkle with feta crumbles for extra saltiness.

HOW IT HELPS YOUR BODY

→ **Fiber:** Lentils and raw vegetables are rich in fiber. This helps regulate bowel function and maintains balanced blood sugar levels, which is essential for stabilizing hormones and energy during menopause.

→ **Omega-3 fatty acids:** The essential fatty acids found in the avocado and flax or chia seeds help support hormonal balance and keep the body's mucous membranes hydrated.

→ **Antioxidants:** Peppers and carrots are rich in vitamins A and C. These vitamins protect cells from free radicals and promote healthy skin and mucous membranes.

→ **Plant protein:** Lentils are a good source of protein, which helps the body maintain muscle mass.

→ **Magnesium:** This mineral found in green vegetables and lentils is essential for stress management and hormonal balance. It also helps relieve cramps and sleep problems associated with menopause.

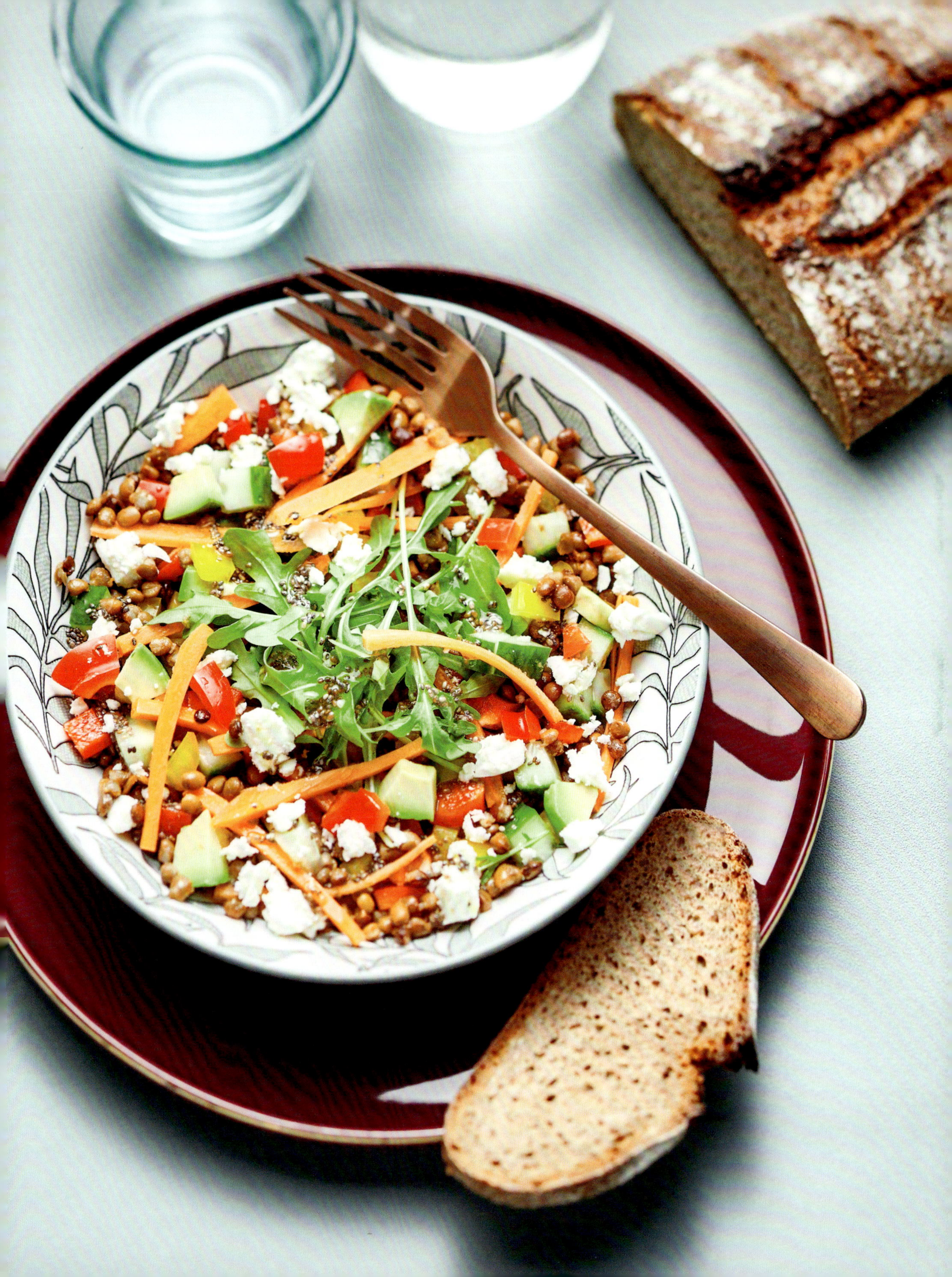

Seaweed Tartare

Serves 4
Soak: 15 minutes
Prep: 15 minutes
Rest: 30 minutes

1.76 oz (50 g) mixture of dried seaweeds (dulse, nori, wakame, etc.)

1 shallot

1 garlic clove

2 tablespoons capers

1 tablespoon lemon juice

1 tablespoon apple cider vinegar

3 tablespoons olive oil

1 tablespoon tamari

1 tablespoon sesame seeds

Pepper, to taste

Fresh parsley

RECIPE

Soak the seaweed in cold water for 10 to 15 minutes. Drain and press to remove any excess water. Peel and thinly slice the shallot and garlic.

Combine the seaweed, capers, shallot, garlic, lemon juice, vinegar, oil, tamari, and sesame seeds. Season with pepper and add chopped parsley before stirring everything together again.

Refrigerate for at least 30 minutes to allow the flavors to develop. Serve the tartare on crackers, sourdough bread, or next to a salad.

HOW IT HELPS YOUR BODY

→ **Iodine:** Seaweed contains iodine, which is essential for a healthy thyroid. Since thyroid function can often be affected during menopause, including iodine in your diet is helpful for regulating metabolism.

→ **Omega-3 fatty acids:** Seaweed and olive oil contain omega-3s that help hydrate the body's mucous membranes, reduce vaginal dryness, and support cardiovascular health.

→ **Antioxidants:** Garlic, shallots, and parsley contain antioxidants that protect cells from oxidative damage and premature aging.

→ **Vitamin C:** Lemon juice and parsley contain vitamin C, which plays a role in collagen production. Collagen is important for maintaining skin elasticity and healthy mucous membranes.

→ **Essential minerals:** Seaweed, tamari, and sesame seeds contain calcium. The magnesium and potassium found in seaweed and sesame seeds are both crucial for bone health, especially during menopause.

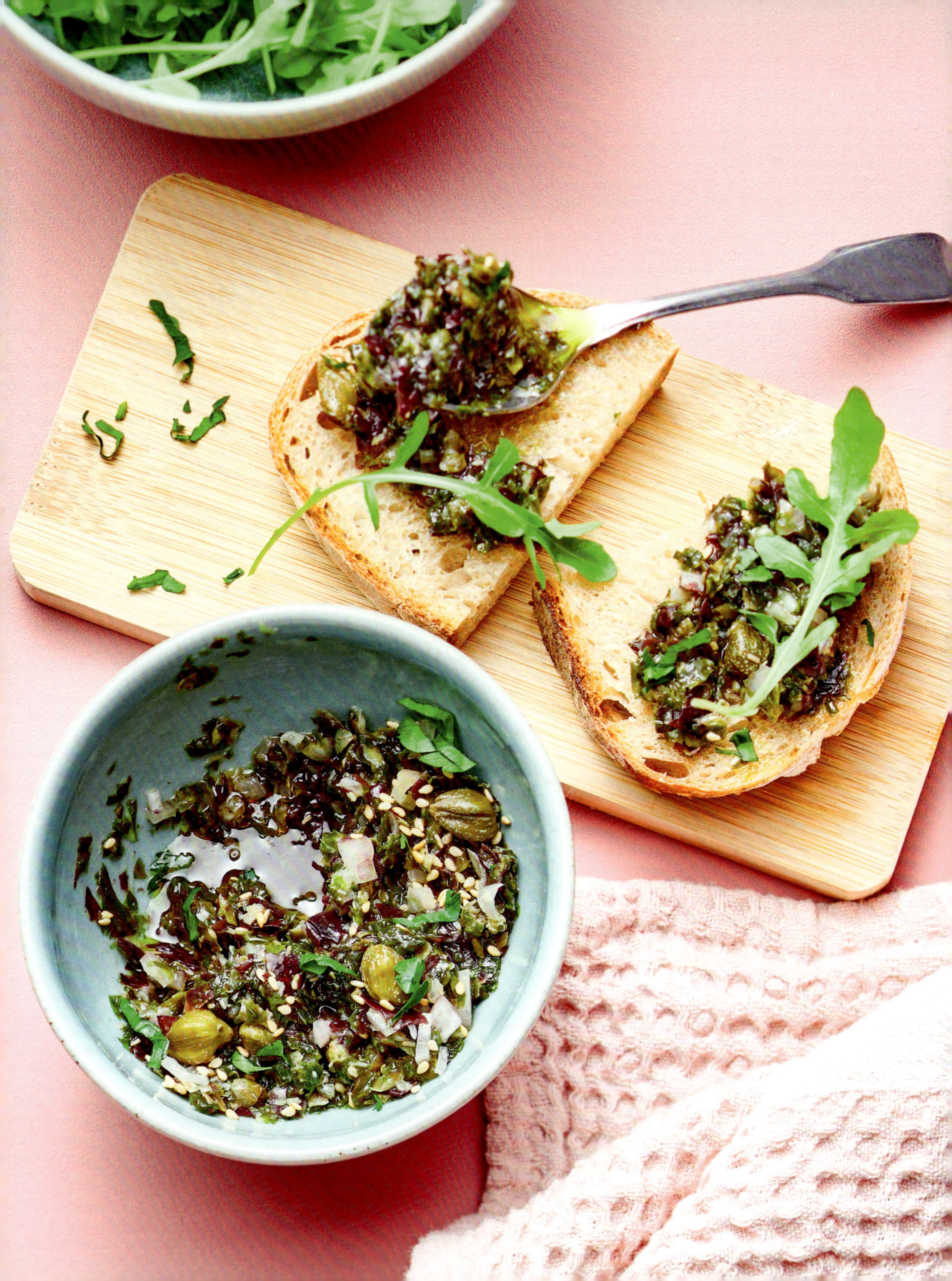

Eggplant Spread

Serves 4
Prep: 10 minutes
Cook: 40 minutes

2 medium eggplants

3 tablespoons olive oil + more for drizzling

2 garlic cloves

Juice of 1 lemon

1 tablespoon tahini

Fresh parsley or cilantro

Pinch ground cumin

Salt and pepper, to taste

RECIPE

Preheat the oven to 400°F (200°C).

Slice the eggplants in half lengthwise and make a few slits in the flesh. Drizzle with olive oil and roast on a baking sheet lined with parchment paper, cut side up, for 30 to 40 minutes until the flesh is tender.

Once the eggplant is cooked, scoop out the flesh with a spoon and mash together with the peeled and chopped garlic, lemon juice, oil, and tahini. Add the chopped herbs and cumin, season with salt and pepper, and stir well. Serve this spread on sourdough bread or with crackers and fresh veggies for dipping.

HOW IT HELPS YOUR BODY

— **Fiber:** Eggplants are rich in fiber, which helps regulate bowel function and maintain stable blood sugar levels.

— **Antioxidants:** The polyphenols found in eggplant skin and the vitamin C in lemons both fight free radicals to ward off cellular aging.

— **Healthy fats:** Olive oil and tahini contain omega-9s and other fatty acids that promote mucous membrane hydration. This can help alleviate the vaginal dryness so often associated with menopause.

— **Vitamin E:** Olive oil contains vitamin E, an antioxidant that helps protect cells and promotes skin regeneration while also supporting healthy mucous membranes.

— **Minerals:** Tahini is rich in calcium, which is essential for bone health, while the fresh herbs add magnesium and potassium to support hormonal balance.

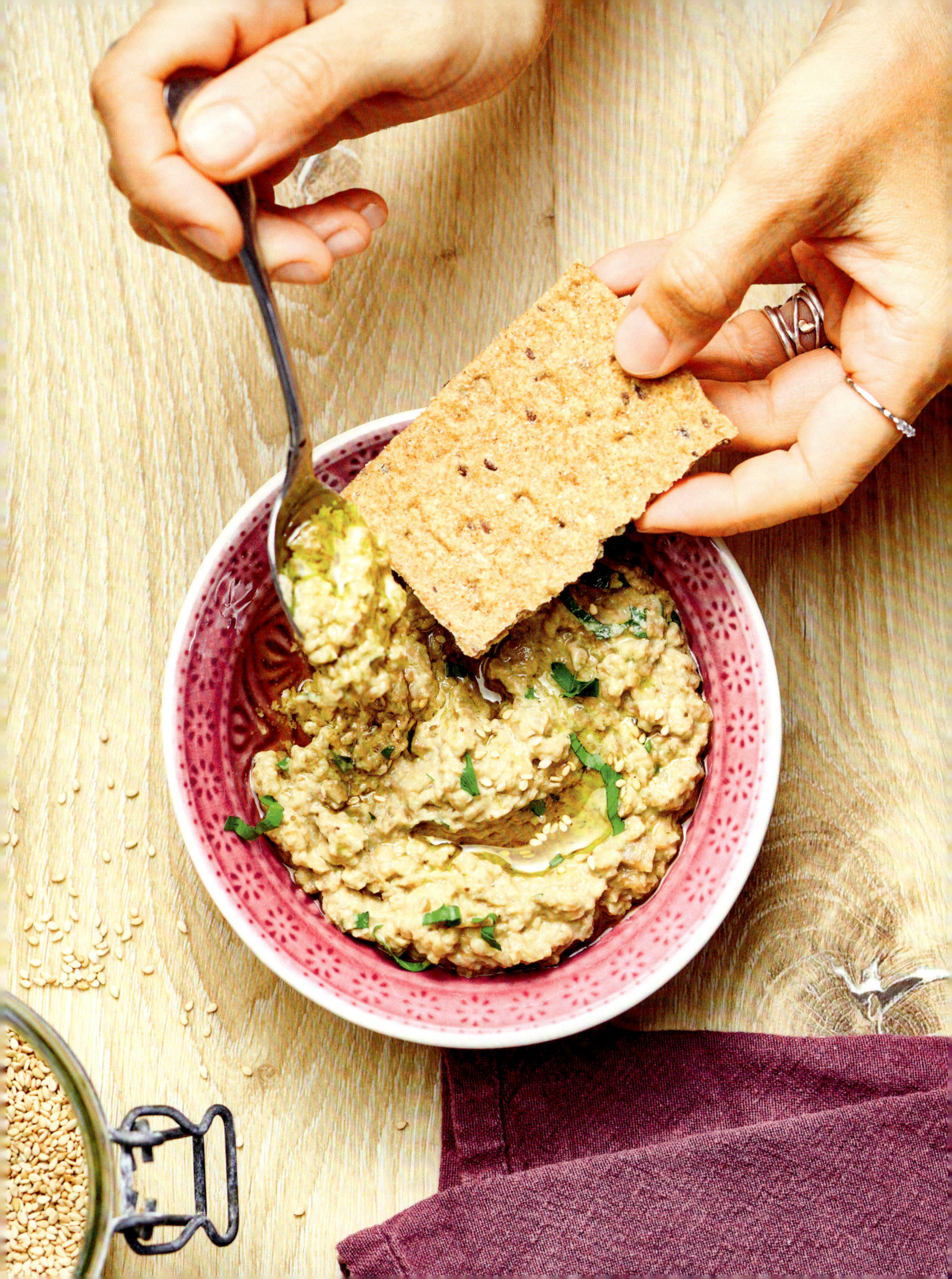

Vegetable Fritters

Serves 4
Prep: 15 minutes
Cook: 10 minutes

2 carrots
2 zucchini
1 onion
1 garlic clove
Handful fresh herbs (parsley, cilantro, or chives)
2 eggs
3 tablespoons chickpea flour
1 tablespoon flaxseed meal
1 tablespoon chia seeds
Salt and pepper, to taste
Pinch turmeric
1 tablespoon olive oil

RECIPE

Peel and grate the carrots and zucchini. Peel the onion and garlic, then thinly slice the onion and press the garlic.

In a bowl, combine the vegetables with the chopped herbs. Beat the eggs and add them to the bowl along with the flour, flaxseed (hydrated in a little water), and chia seeds. Stir until combined. Season with salt and pepper and add the turmeric.

Use your hands or a spoon to shape the batter into small patties. Heat the oil in a pan over medium heat. Fry the fritters for around 5 minutes on each side until they are golden and crispy. Serve hot alongside a green salad or with a seasoned sheep's milk yogurt sauce for added freshness.

HOW IT HELPS YOUR BODY

→ **Fiber:** Carrots and zucchini are rich in fiber; which helps maintain regular bowel function and healthy blood sugar levels.

→ **Protein:** Eggs, chia seeds, and chickpea flour all contain protein that is essential for tissue repair and preventing muscle loss.

→ **Omega-3 fatty acids:** The omega-3s in flaxseed and chia seeds help balance hormones and hydrate the body's mucous membranes.

→ **Antioxidants:** Carrots are rich in beta-carotene, a vitamin A precursor that is useful for keeping skin and tissues hydrated.

→ **B vitamins:** Chickpeas and eggs contain B vitamins that play an essential role in energy production and nervous system support. They also help reduce fatigue.

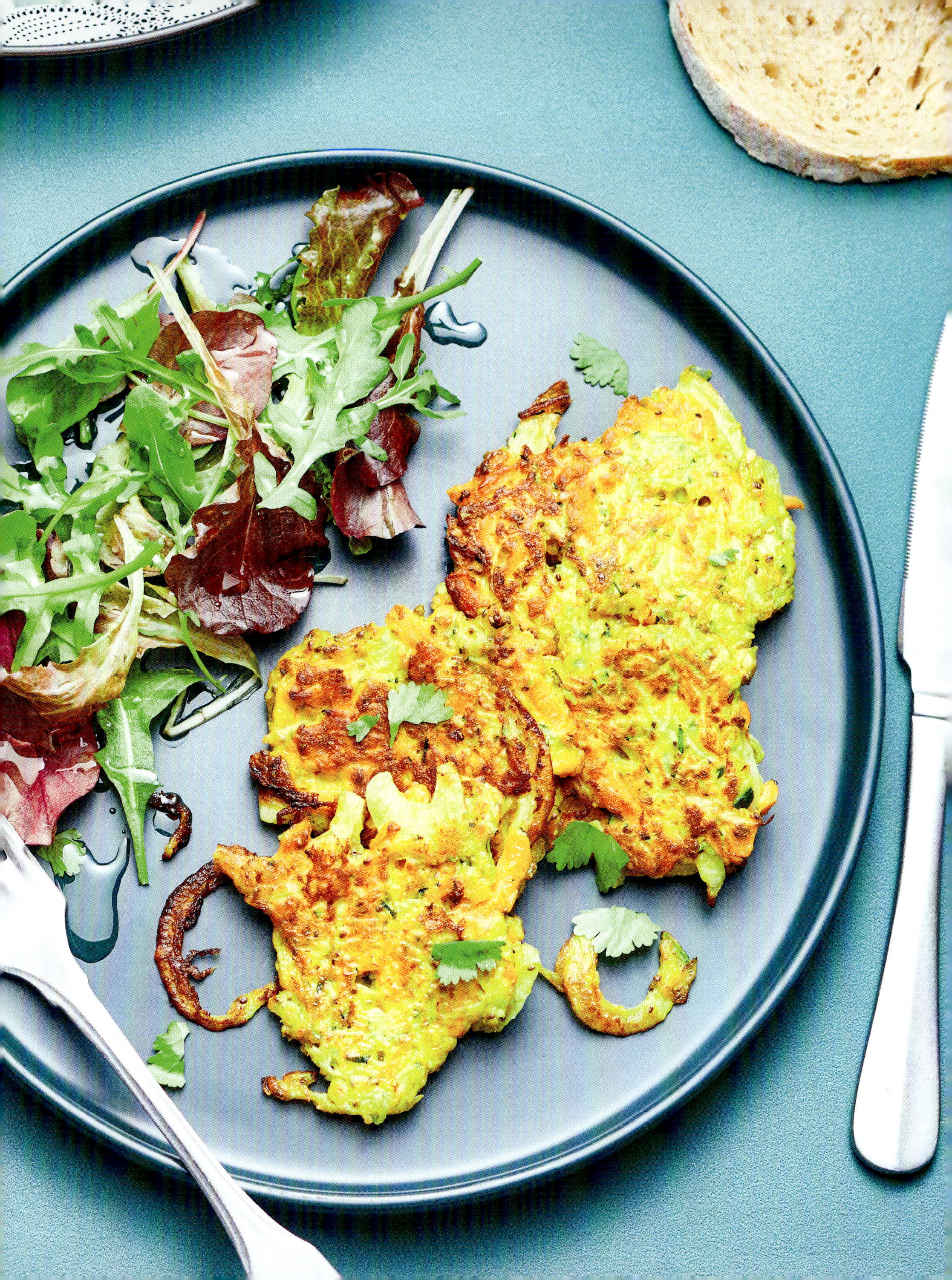

Roasted Chicken and Sweet Potatoes

Serves 4
Prep: 15 minutes
Cook: 1 hour 15 minutes
Rest: 10 minutes

1 whole chicken (around 2.6 pounds [1.2 kg])

2 tablespoons olive oil

Salt and pepper, to taste

2 garlic cloves

1 tablespoon fresh thyme

1 tablespoon fresh rosemary

1 organic lemon

1 red onion

4 medium sweet potatoes

1 tablespoon flaxseed oil

Handful fresh spinach

1 tablespoon pumpkin seeds

RECIPE

Preheat the oven to 400°F (200°C).

Rub the chicken with olive oil, salt, pepper, peeled and crushed garlic, thyme, and rosemary. Cut the lemon in half and place both halves inside the chicken cavity. Place the chicken in a baking tray. Peel and quarter the onion and arrange the quarters around the chicken.

Peel the sweet potatoes and cut into pieces. Rub with oil and season with salt and pepper. Arrange the sweet potato pieces around the chicken.

Bake for around 1 hour and 15 minutes, basting the chicken with its own juices every 20 minutes. Check for doneness by poking the thigh: The juices should be clear. If necessary, continue cooking for 10 extra minutes. Once the chicken is cooked, let it rest for 10 minutes before slicing.

Before serving the chicken, drizzle a little flaxseed oil over the sweet potatoes, add the spinach, and scatter with pumpkin seeds for an extra crunch.

HOW IT HELPS YOUR BODY

Protein: Chicken contains protein, which is essential for maintaining muscle mass. It also plays a role in cell regeneration.

Beta-carotene: Sweet potatoes contain beta-carotene. This vitamin A precursor is a powerful antioxidant that supports healthy tissue and skin.

Zinc: Pumpkin seeds contain zinc, which plays a key role in hormonal health and tissue repair. It is also essential for healthy immunity.

Omega-3 fatty acids: Flaxseed oil contains omega-3s that support hormone production, help fight against inflammation, and keep mucous membranes flexible.

Fiber: Sweet potatoes and spinach contain fiber, which promotes healthy digestion and bowel function.

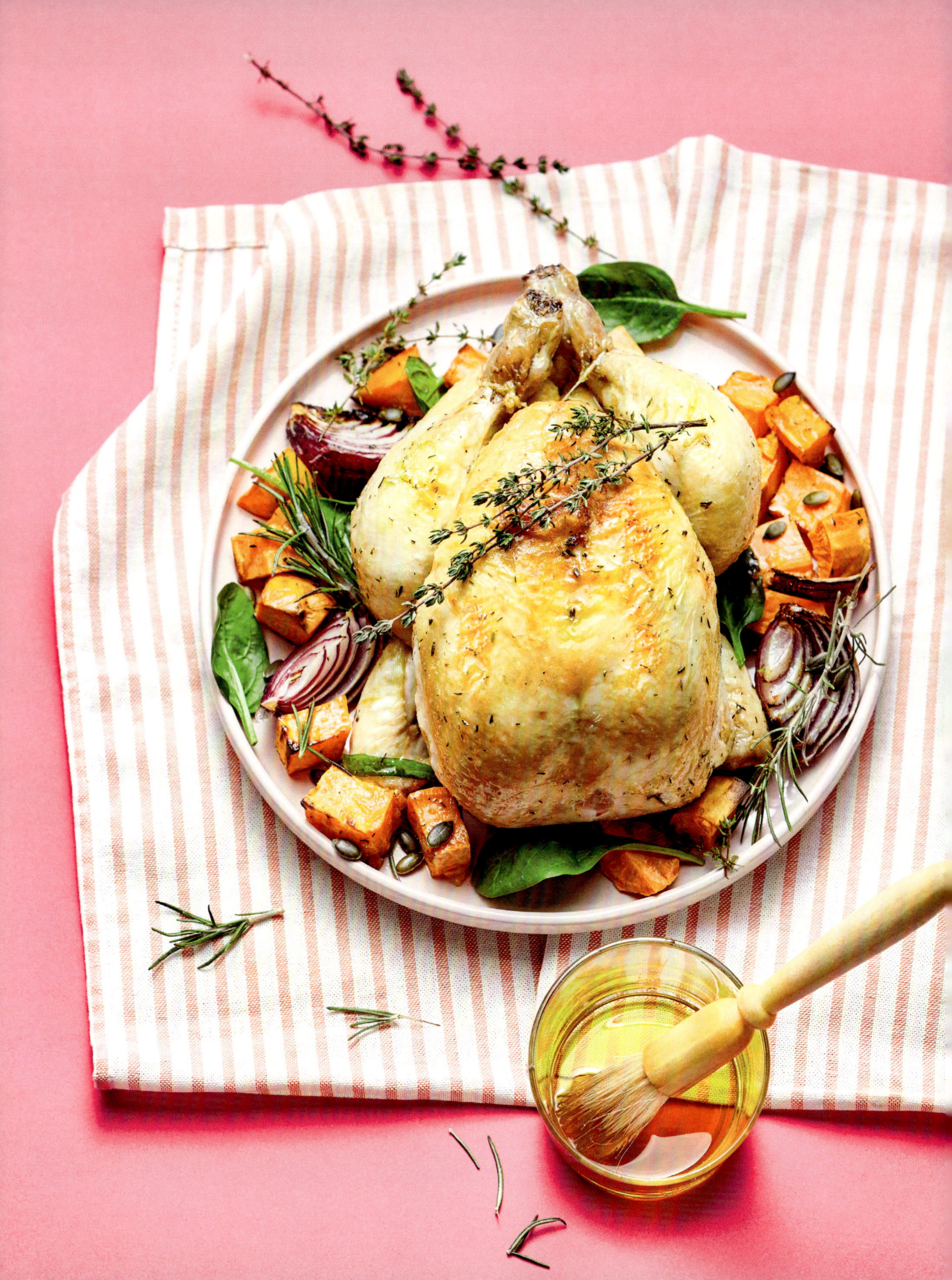

Recipes for Better Sleep

Our sleep routines are often thrown off during menopause, usually as a result of hot flashes or increased stress. Foods containing magnesium, tryptophan, and complex carbohydrates promote relaxation and melatonin production for a restorative night's sleep.

Tryptophan

Tryptophan

Tryptophan is an essential amino acid, which means that our bodies cannot produce it and we can only get it from the food we eat. It is a key part of serotonin and melatonin synthesis. These two neurotransmitters (we'll be referring to them as hormones, too) are critical for mood regulation, sleep, and overall well-being.

Serotonin

In the brain, tryptophan is converted into 5-hydroxytryptophan (5-HTP), which is then transformed into serotonin. Serotonin is often called the "happiness hormone" because it plays such an important role in managing mood, anxiety, and stress. Healthy levels of serotonin promote relaxation and a sense of calm, both of which are essential for managing menopause symptoms like mood swings and irritability.

Melatonin

Once serotonin is produced, it is used to make melatonin, the hormone that regulates our wake-sleep cycle. Melatonin is naturally secreted when the sun goes down and signals the body that it is time to rest. During menopause, hormonal fluctuations and especially the drop in estrogen levels can disrupt melatonin production and cause sleep problems. Tryptophan therefore plays a crucial role in safeguarding the body's restorative sleep.

Tryptophan
→ 5-hydroxytryptophan
→ Serotonin
→ Melatonin

Foods Rich in Tryptophan

Grains and beans
Split peas, oat bran, red beans, lentils, whole wheat, whole-grain rice

Seeds and nuts
Sesame seeds, walnuts, almonds, cashews

Fruit
Pineapple, avocado, banana, fig, raisins, dates, kiwi

Fish and shellfish
Cod, lobster, tuna

Cheeses
Parmesan, Gruyère, Gouda

Meat and eggs
Roasted chicken with the skin on, steak, turkey, rabbit

Other
Raw cacao

Magnesium

Magnesium (see page 30) is one of the most important minerals for overall health. It plays a role in more than 300 enzymatic reactions and regulates many of the body's functions from blood pressure to nervous system and muscle function.

Muscle and nerve relaxation

Magnesium acts as a natural relaxant and helps to calm the nervous system and relax the muscles. This makes it a crucial part of battling sleep problems that often arise during menopause when hot flashes, night sweats, and stress keep you up at night. By making it easier for the body to relax and reducing stress, magnesium can help improve sleep quality.

Anti-inflammatory effects and stress management

Magnesium is also a powerful anti-inflammatory. During menopause, many women experience increased inflammation and joint pain, partly due to the drop in estrogen levels. Getting enough magnesium can help reduce inflammation and ease physical discomfort. What's more, it helps modulate the body's response to stress by lowering cortisol (a stress hormone) and stabilizing mood.

Hormonal benefits

Decreased estrogen levels can lead to a variety of symptoms like fatigue, weight gain, and mood swings. Magnesium helps rebalance hormones and contributes to energy production, which can help reduce fatigue. It is also helpful for bone health and works together with calcium and vitamin D at the time in a woman's life when she is most at risk for developing osteoporosis.

Foods Rich in Magnesium

Green vegetables
Broccoli, kale, cabbage, spinach, Swiss chard, lettuce, arugula, lamb's lettuce

Fatty fish
Sardine, mackerel, wild salmon, herring, wild tuna, anchovies

Fruit
Avocado, banana, fig, raisin, dates, kiwi

Whole grains
Quinoa, oat, brown rice, buckwheat, barley, millet

Nuts and seeds
Almonds, pumpkin seeds, sesame seeds, cashews, Brazil nuts, flaxseed, chia seeds, sunflower seeds

Beans
Black beans, white beans, lentils, chickpeas, edamame

Other
Dark chocolate, tofu, nutritional yeast, wheat germ

Marseille Fish Soup

Serves 4
Prep: 20 minutes
Cook: 35 minutes

1 onion

2 garlic cloves

1 red bell pepper, seeds removed

1 fennel bulb

2 tomatoes

2 tablespoons olive oil

1 tablespoon tomato paste

Pinch saffron

1 teaspoon turmeric

1 teaspoon smoked paprika

1 quart (1 l) vegetable or fish broth, unsalted

17.6 ounces (500 g) whitefish fillets (hake, cod, or pollock)

7 ounces (200 g) shrimp, peeled and deveined

Juice of 1 lemon

Salt and pepper, to taste

Fresh parsley or cilantro

RECIPE

Peel the onion and garlic. Thinly slice the onion, garlic, pepper, and fennel. Cut the tomatoes into cubes.

Heat the oil in a large pot and add the onion, garlic, pepper and fennel. Cook for around 5 minutes until tender. Add the tomatoes and tomato paste. Cook for another 5 minutes. Add the saffron, turmeric, and paprika. Stir well. Pour in the broth, bring to a boil, then lower the heat and cook for 15 minutes.

Cut the fish fillets into pieces and add to the soup along with the shrimp. Let cook for 10 more minutes until the fish is nice and tender. Add the lemon juice and season with salt and pepper.

Top the soup with parsley or cilantro just before serving with whole-grain toast or garlic-rubbed croutons for a balanced meal.

HOW IT HELPS YOUR BODY

- **Tryptophan and magnesium:** Whitefish and shrimp are sources of tryptophan, an amino acid precursor to serotonin and melatonin that promotes restorative sleep. These ingredients are also rich in magnesium, which is essential for muscle relaxation and reducing stress.
- **Omega-3 fatty acids:** Whitefish contains omega-3s that help regulate inflammation and support hormonal health.
- **Antioxidants:** The vegetables in this soup are rich in antioxidants (in particular vitamin C) that protect cells from oxidative stress and promote healthy skin tissue.
- **Fiber and digestion:** Vegetables are a good source of fiber and promote healthy digestion while also stabilizing blood glucose levels. This is important for quality sleep and hormonal balance.
- **Anti-inflammatory effects:** Turmeric and paprika are known for their anti-inflammatory and antioxidant properties. They support overall comfort during menopause in addition to contributing to nervous system health.

Split Pea Soup

Serves 4
Prep: 10 minutes
Cook: 50 minutes

8.8 ounces (250 g) split peas

1 onion

2 garlic cloves

2 carrots

1 leek

1 celery stalk

1 tablespoon olive oil

1 bay leaf

1 teaspoon thyme

1 teaspoon ground cumin

1.5 quarts (1.5 l) vegetable broth, unsalted

Salt and pepper, to taste

Juice of ½ lemon

Fresh parsley or cilantro

RECIPE

Rinse the split peas under cold water until the water runs clear. Drain thoroughly. Peel the onion, garlic, and carrots and thinly slice. Thinly slice the leek and celery.

Heat the olive oil in a large pot over medium heat. Add the onion, garlic, leek, carrots, and celery. Cook for 5 to 7 minutes until tender. Add the split peas, bay leaf, thyme, and cumin.

Pour in the broth, bring to a boil, then lower the heat and cook, covered, for 40 to 45 minutes until the split peas are tender. Stir occasionally.

Once the split peas are cooked, remove the bay leaf. If you want a smooth, velvety texture you can blend the soup. Otherwise, just leave it as is.

Season with salt and pepper and add a drizzle of lemon juice before serving hot topped with chopped parsley or cilantro. You can serve this soup with sourdough bread on the side for a balanced meal.

HOW IT HELPS YOUR BODY

Plant protein and tryptophan: Split peas are rich in plant protein, which is essential for maintaining muscle mass. They also contain tryptophan, an amino acid that promotes serotonin production. Serotonin improves mood and sleep quality.

Magnesium: Split peas and other vegetables in this recipe contain magnesium, a key mineral for reducing stress, relaxing muscles, and promoting better sleep.

Fiber and blood sugar control: This soup is rich in fiber (split peas, carrots, celery), which helps regulate digestion and stabilize blood sugar. This makes it easier to manage hormonal fluctuations and prevent insulin spikes that can disturb sleep.

Antioxidants and cardiovascular health: Carrots and leeks are rich in antioxidants like vitamin A and vitamin C that protect cells from aging. Garlic contributes to cardiovascular health.

Calming + anti-inflammatory: Cumin and thyme both have natural anti-inflammatory properties that help relieve inflammation symptoms and calm the body. This in turn promotes better sleep.

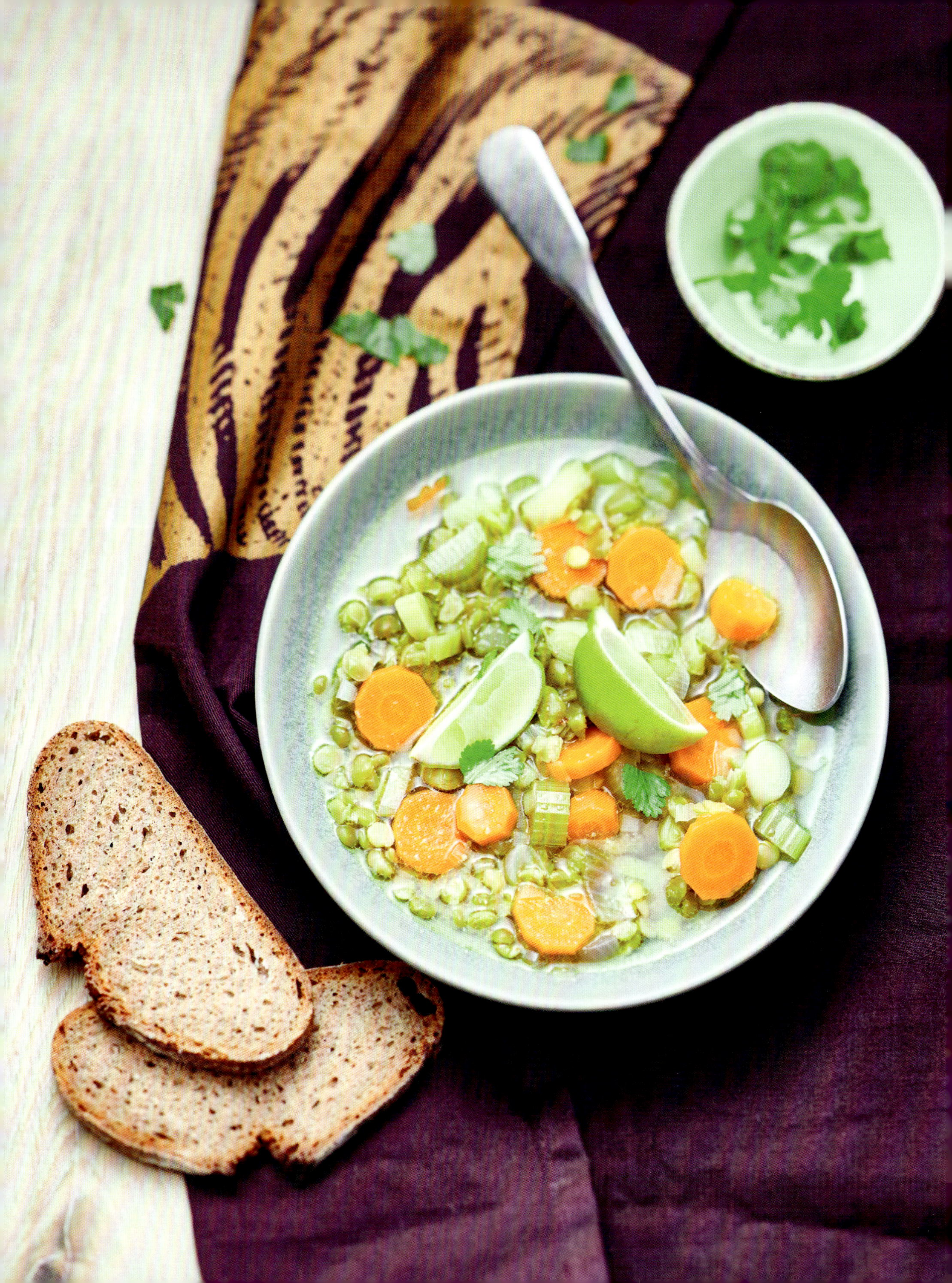

Black Bean Vegetarian Chili

Serves 4
Prep: 15 minutes
Cook: 30 minutes

1 red onion
2 garlic cloves
1 red bell pepper
1 yellow bell pepper
1 small red chili pepper (optional)
1 tablespoon olive oil
1 teaspoon ground cumin
1 teaspoon smoked paprika
1 teaspoon turmeric
14 ounces (400 g) crushed tomatoes
1 tablespoon tomato paste
1 teaspoon tamari
14 ounces (400 g) cooked black beans
5.3 ounces (150 g) corn kernels (canned)
1 tablespoon unsweetened cacao powder (optional)
Salt and pepper, to taste
Juice of 1 lime
Fresh cilantro

RECIPE

Peel the onion and garlic. Thinly slice the onion, garlic, peppers, and chili pepper if using.

Heat the oil in a large pan or Dutch oven over medium heat. Cook the onion, garlic, and peppers for around 5 minutes until tender. Add the cumin, paprika, and turmeric. Stir well. Add the tomatoes, tomato paste, and tamari. Cook for 10 minutes over low heat.

Add the beans, corn, and cacao (if using) then cook for another 10 to 15 minutes over low heat. Add salt and pepper as needed.

Drizzle with lime juice and sprinkle with chopped cilantro before serving. For a balanced meal, serve this chili with whole-grain rice and a green salad.

HOW IT HELPS YOUR BODY

- **Tryptophan and magnesium:** Black beans and corn are both sources of tryptophan, an amino acid that is necessary for the production of serotonin. Serotonin regulates mood and promotes healthy sleep. They also contain magnesium, which is essential for muscle and nervous system relaxation and helps reduce stress and improve sleep.
- **Fiber and digestive health:** Black beans are rich in fiber and promote healthy digestion and blood sugar control.
- **Antioxidants:** Peppers and tomatoes are rich in vitamin C and antioxidants, which protect cells from premature aging. Cacao is rich in flavonoids and also contributes to cardiovascular health.
- **Anti-inflammation:** Spices are known for their natural anti-inflammatory properties and reduce inflammation as well as joint and muscle pain.

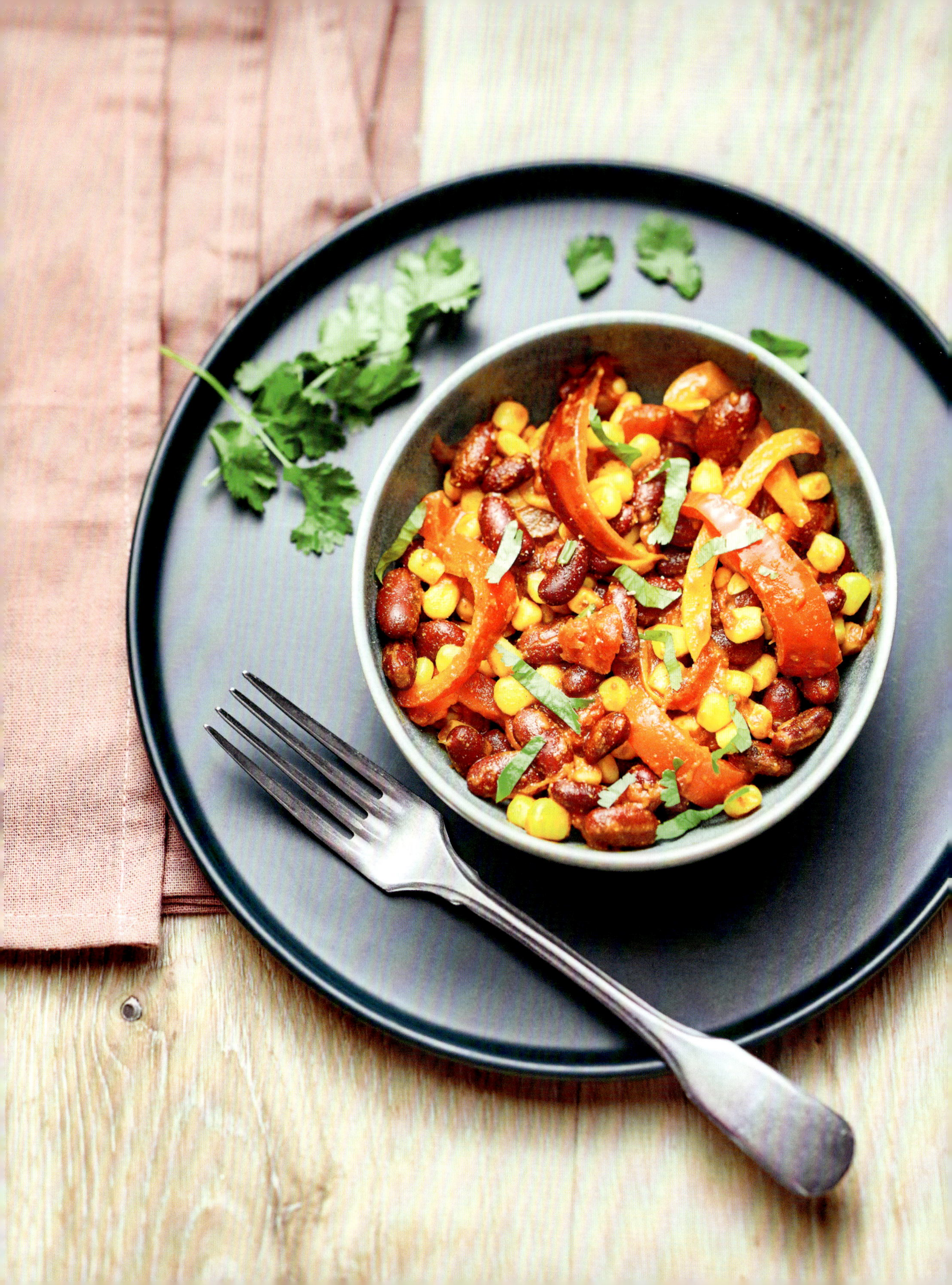

Steamed Fish and Vegetables with Whole-Grain Rice

Serves 4
Prep: 20 minutes
Cook: 30 minutes

7 ounces (200 g) whole-grain rice

2 carrots

1 zucchini

1 red bell pepper

1 head broccoli

4 whitefish fillets (cod, pollock, or hake)

1 tablespoon tamari

1 tablespoon lemon juice

1 tablespoon sesame oil

1 tablespoon fresh ginger, grated

1 garlic clove

2 tablespoons sesame seeds, toasted

Fresh cilantro

Mixed greens (optional)

RECIPE

Rinse the rice under cold water until the water runs clear. Cook for around 30 minutes in a pot of salted boiling water, following the instructions on the packet, until the rice is tender. Drain.

Peel the carrots then cut the carrots, zucchini, and pepper into thin matchsticks. Chop the broccoli into small florets (feel free to add other seasonal vegetables). Steam for 8 to 10 minutes—they should be tender crisp and still have a little bit of bite to them.

While the vegetables are steaming, steam the fish for 10 minutes.

Combine the tamari, lemon juice, oil, ginger, and garlic (peeled and minced).

Divide the rice between 4 plates. Top with vegetables and fish. Pour over the sauce and sprinkle with toasted sesame seeds and cilantro. Serve hot with a green salad on the side if desired.

HOW IT HELPS YOUR BODY

Tryptophan and magnesium: Whole-grain rice is rich in tryptophan, an amino acid that promotes serotonin and melatonin production to help the body regulate sleep. Fish is an excellent source of magnesium, which helps muscles relax and reduces stress.

Omega-3 fatty acids: Whitefish is a source of lean protein and contains omega-3 fatty acids, which support cardiovascular health and help regulate inflammation and hormones.

Fiber: The fiber found in whole-grain rice and the vegetables in this recipe helps maintain healthy digestion and stabilizes blood sugar levels, all of which promotes better sleep.

Antioxidants: Red peppers and broccoli are rich in antioxidants like vitamins C and E that help protect skin and tissue cells from oxidative stress.

B vitamins and calcium: B vitamins (fish and whole-grain rice) and calcium (green vegetables) are essential for muscle and nervous system equilibrium. They also promote relaxation and healthy sleep.

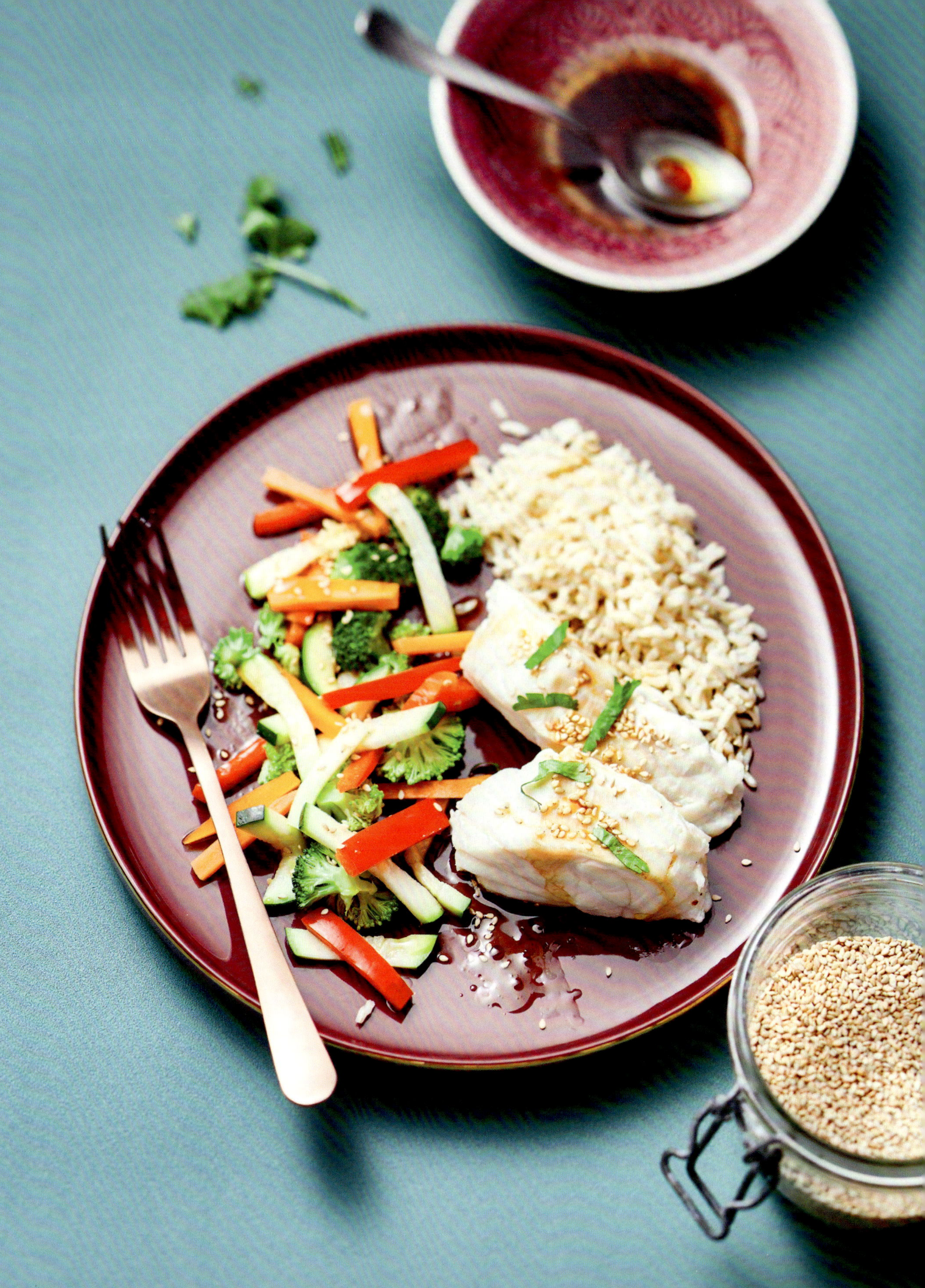

Banana-Chocolate Protein Smoothie

Serves 1
Prep: 10 minutes

1 ripe banana

2 tablespoons lupine flour

2 tablespoons raw cacao powder

8 fluid ounces (250 ml) almond milk (or other plant-based milk)

1 tablespoon chia seeds

RECIPE

Peel the banana and cut into pieces.

Add the banana pieces, lupine flour, cacao, milk, and chia seeds to a blender. Blend until smooth, pour into a glass, and serve.

HOW IT HELPS YOUR BODY

- **Protein:** Lupine flour is rich in protein, which is essential for maintaining muscle mass and helps with tissue regeneration.
- **Magnesium:** The magnesium in the chia seeds and almond milk helps reduce stress and improves sleep quality.
- **Tryptophan:** Banana and cacao contain tryptophan, an amino acid precursor to serotonin. Tryptophan is also important in the production of melatonin, a sleep-regulating hormone that can improve sleep quality.
- **Antioxidants:** Raw cacao is rich in antioxidants that help combat oxidative stress and inflammation to boost overall well-being.
- **Fiber:** Chia seeds and bananas contain fiber, which supports healthy digestion and may help you avoid digestive issues.

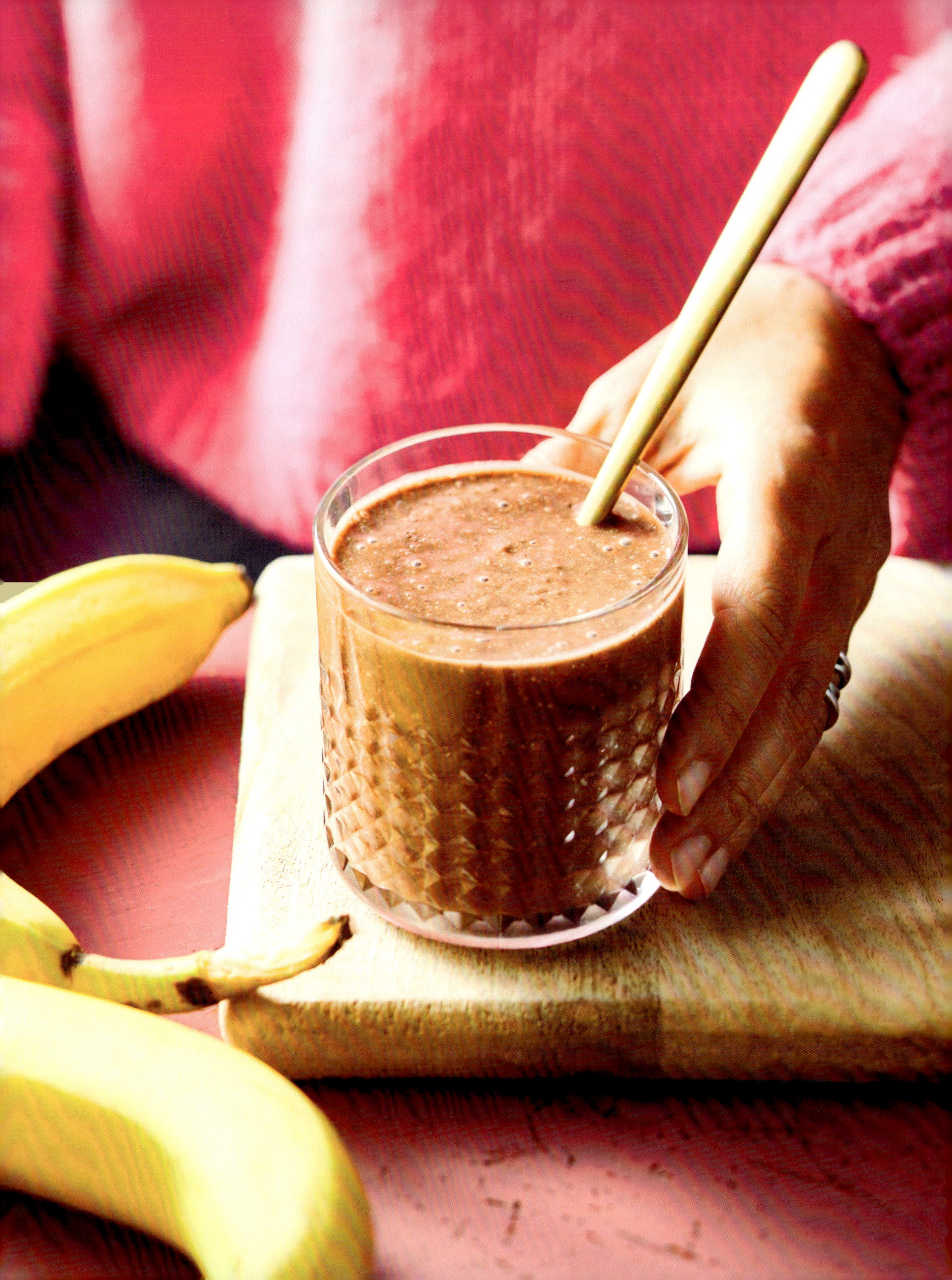

Dark Chocolate Crunchy Quinoa Bites

Makes 12 bites
Prep: 15 minutes
Refrigeration: 30 minutes

3.5 ounces (100 g) raw quinoa

5.3 ounces (150 g) raw dark chocolate (at least 70 percent cacao)

1 tablespoon coconut oil

2 tablespoons chia seeds

2 tablespoons sesame seeds

Pinch salt

RECIPE

Toast the raw quinoa for 3 to 5 minutes in a pan over medium until crunchy.

Melt the chocolate with the coconut oil in a water bath. Add the chia seeds, sesame seeds, crunchy quinoa, and salt. Stir well.

Use a spoon to make 12 small mounds on a baking sheet lined with parchment paper. Refrigerate for 30 minutes until the bites harden. Serve them straight out of the refrigerator to preserve their texture.

HOW IT HELPS YOUR BODY

- **Magnesium:** Raw dark chocolate is rich in magnesium, which is essential for muscle relaxation and stress management. It also ensures good sleep.
- **Omega-3 fatty acids:** Chia seeds are a source of omega-3s, which help regulate inflammation and contribute to hormonal health.
- **Antioxidants:** Raw dark chocolate is rich in antioxidants, which protect cells from oxidative stress and can help prevent premature aging.
- **Fiber:** The fiber in this recipe (quinoa and seeds) promotes healthy digestion. It also helps regulate blood sugar levels.
- **Vitamin E:** Vitamin E (coconut oil, sesame seeds) is a fat-soluble antioxidant that supports healthy skin and helps maintain hydration in the body. This is helpful for battling common menopause symptoms like vaginal dryness.

TIP

You can add berries (cranberries, goji berries . . .) or chopped nuts (walnuts, hazelnuts, almonds) to this recipe for extra crunch and nutrients.

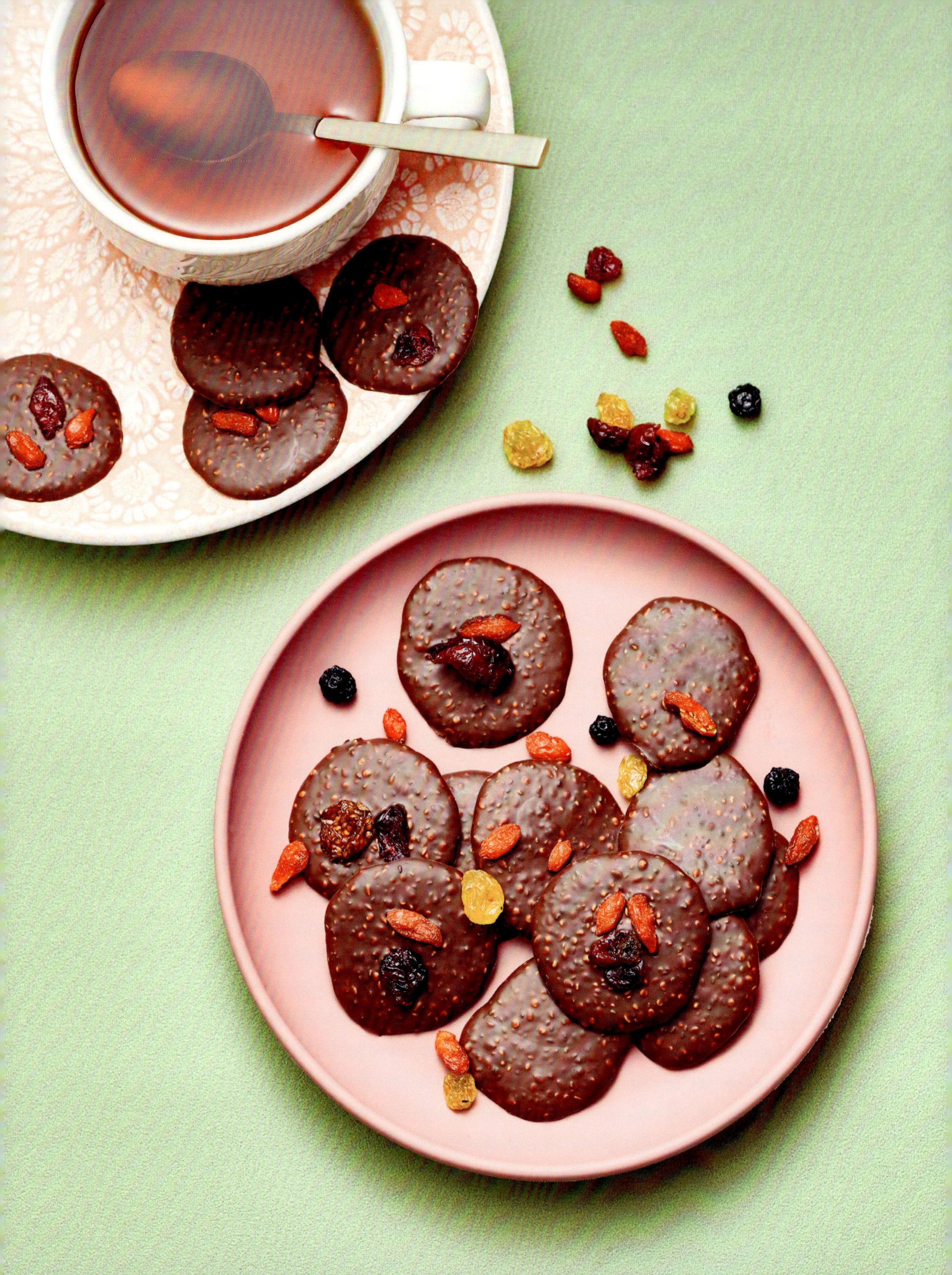

Cashew Ice Cream

Serves 4
Soak: 4 hours
Prep: 10 minutes
Freeze: 4 hours

7 ounces (200 g) cashews

8 fluid ounces (250 ml) almond milk (or other plant-based milk)

3 tablespoons maple syrup (or other natural sweetener)

1 teaspoon vanilla extract

2 tablespoons chia seeds

Pinch salt

Handful berries, fresh or frozen

RECIPE

Soak the cashews for at least 4 hours or overnight. Drain and rinse under cold water.

Add the cashews, almond milk, maple syrup, vanilla, chia seeds, and salt to a blender. Blend until smooth and creamy. Add berries and blend until smooth.

Pour the mixture into a freezer-safe container and let set for 4 hours until firm, stirring every 30 minutes for the first few hours to prevent crystals from forming. Remove the ice cream from the freezer around 5 minutes before you plan to eat it to make it easier to serve.

HOW IT HELPS YOUR BODY

Protein and healthy fats: Cashews are an excellent source of protein and healthy fats, which are necessary for maintaining hormonal balance and promoting healthy skin. They also contain unsaturated fatty acids that can help reduce inflammation.

Magnesium: Cashews are rich in magnesium, an essential mineral that helps regulate stress and improve sleep quality.

Tryptophan: Almond milk and cashews contain tryptophan, an amino acid serotonin precursor that plays an important role in mood and sleep regulation.

Fiber: Chia seeds contain fiber. This promotes healthy digestion and contributes to blood sugar level regulation, which is important for maintaining energy and preventing sudden cravings.

Antioxidants: Berries are rich in antioxidants, which help combat oxidative stress and inflammation.

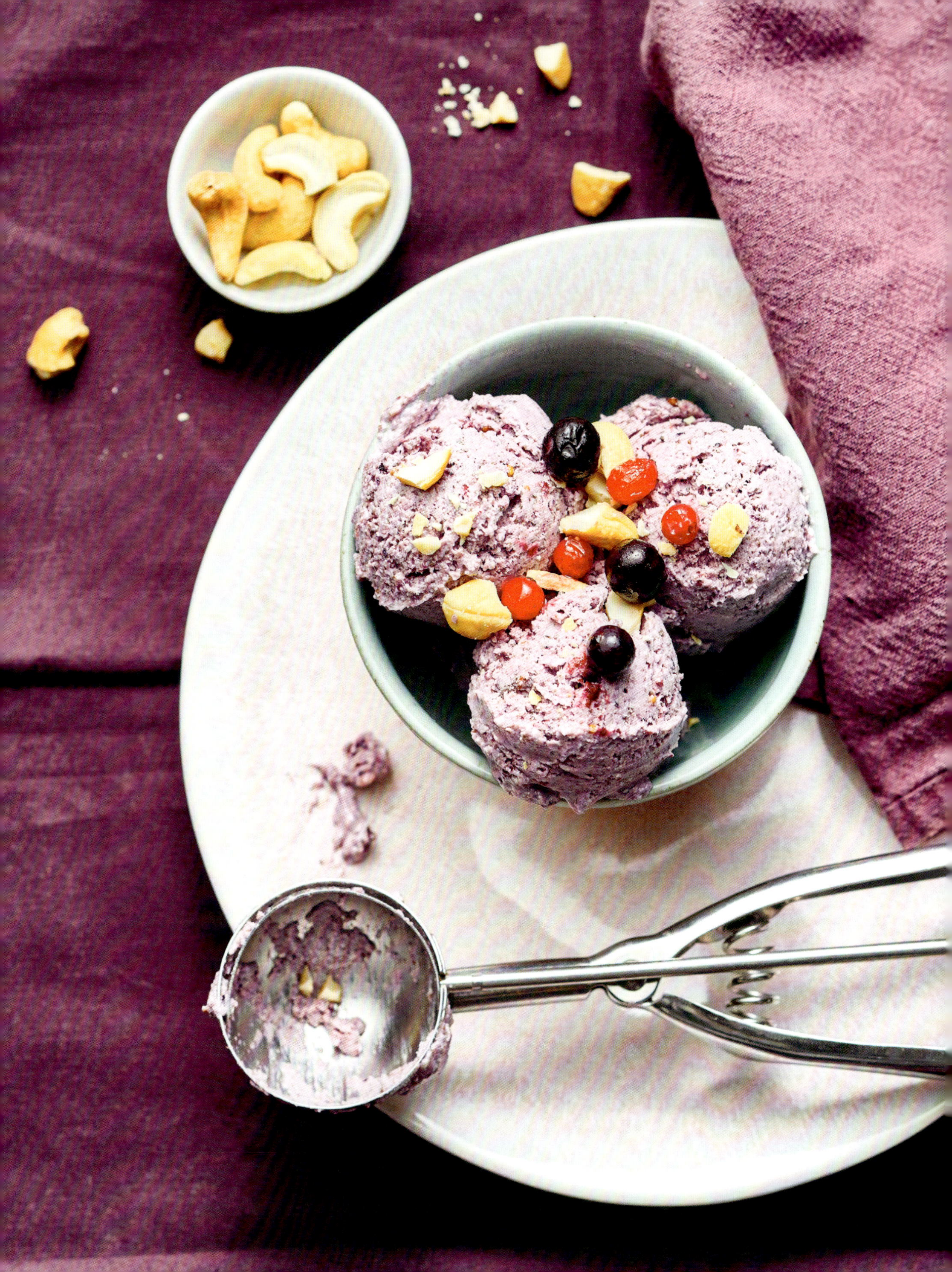

Cacao-Coconut Energy Balls

Makes 12 energy balls
Soak: 10 minutes
Prep: 15 minutes
Refrigeration: 30 minutes

5.3 ounces (150 g) dates, pitted

3.5 ounces (100 g) cashews

1.76 ounces (50 g) coconut flakes

1 ounce (30 g) raw cacao powder

1 tablespoon chia seeds

Pinch salt

RECIPE

Soak the dates in lukewarm water for 10 minutes to soften them. Drain thoroughly.

Use a food processor or blender to blend the cashews into a fine powder. Add the drained dates and blend until combined. Add the coconut, cacao powder, chia seeds, and salt. Blend again until combined. If the mixture is too dry, add 1 to 2 tablespoons of water to loosen it.

Use your hands to form walnut-size balls. Then, if you want a tasty outer layer, roll each ball in coconut flakes until coated.

Transfer the energy balls to a baking sheet lined with parchment paper and refrigerate for at least 30 minutes before serving so they have time to firm up.

HOW IT HELPS YOUR BODY

- **Magnesium:** This mineral is found in cashews and chia seeds. It helps regulate stress and improves sleep by promoting muscle and nervous system relaxation.
- **Tryptophan:** Found in cashews and chia seeds, tryptophan is an essential amino acid that helps produce serotonin. Serotonin is a neurotransmitter that is important for regulating mood and the sleep cycle.
- **Fiber:** Dates, cashews, and chia seeds are rich in fiber, which helps maintain digestive health and stabilizes blood sugar levels. This contributes to better mood regulation.
- **Antioxidants:** Raw cacao and coconut contain antioxidants that combat oxidative stress and help protect cells.
- **Omega-3 fatty acids:** Chia seeds are rich in omega-3 fatty acids, which are beneficial for heart health and maintaining hormonal balance.

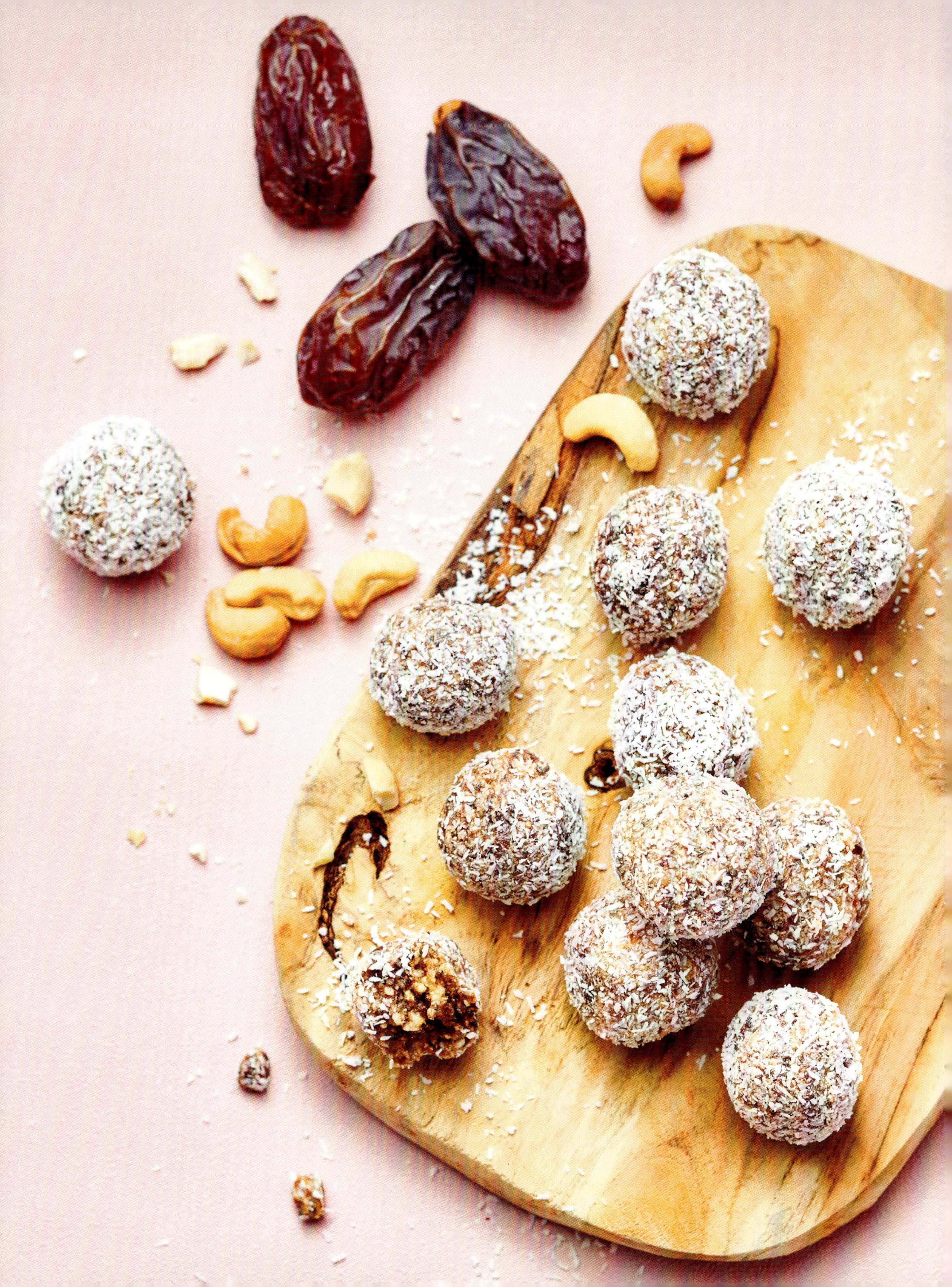

Six Healthy Snacks for Better Sleep

Serves 1
Prep: 5 minutes

Avocado-strawberry salad

1 avocado • 5.3 ounces (150 g) strawberries • 1 tablespoon pumpkin seeds

Cut the avocado and strawberries into pieces. Combine with the pumpkin seeds. Season with a little lemon juice.

Bananas and almond butter

1 banana • 2 tablespoons almond butter

Peel and slice the banana. Spread a thin layer of almond butter on each slice. Serve immediately.

Almonds and pear slices

Handful almonds • 1 pear

Slice the pear and enjoy with a handful of almonds.

Chocolate and cashews

1 ounce (30 g) dark chocolate 70 percent cacao • Handful cashews

Break the chocolate into small pieces and serve with the cashews.

Banana oat smoothie

1 peeled banana • ¼ cup oatmeal • 1 cup almond milk

Blend ingredients until smooth. Serve chilled.

Avocado toast with pumpkin seeds

1 avocado • 1 slice of whole-grain bread, toasted • 1 tablespoon pumpkin seeds

Smash the avocado onto the slice of bread. Sprinkle with pumpkin seeds.

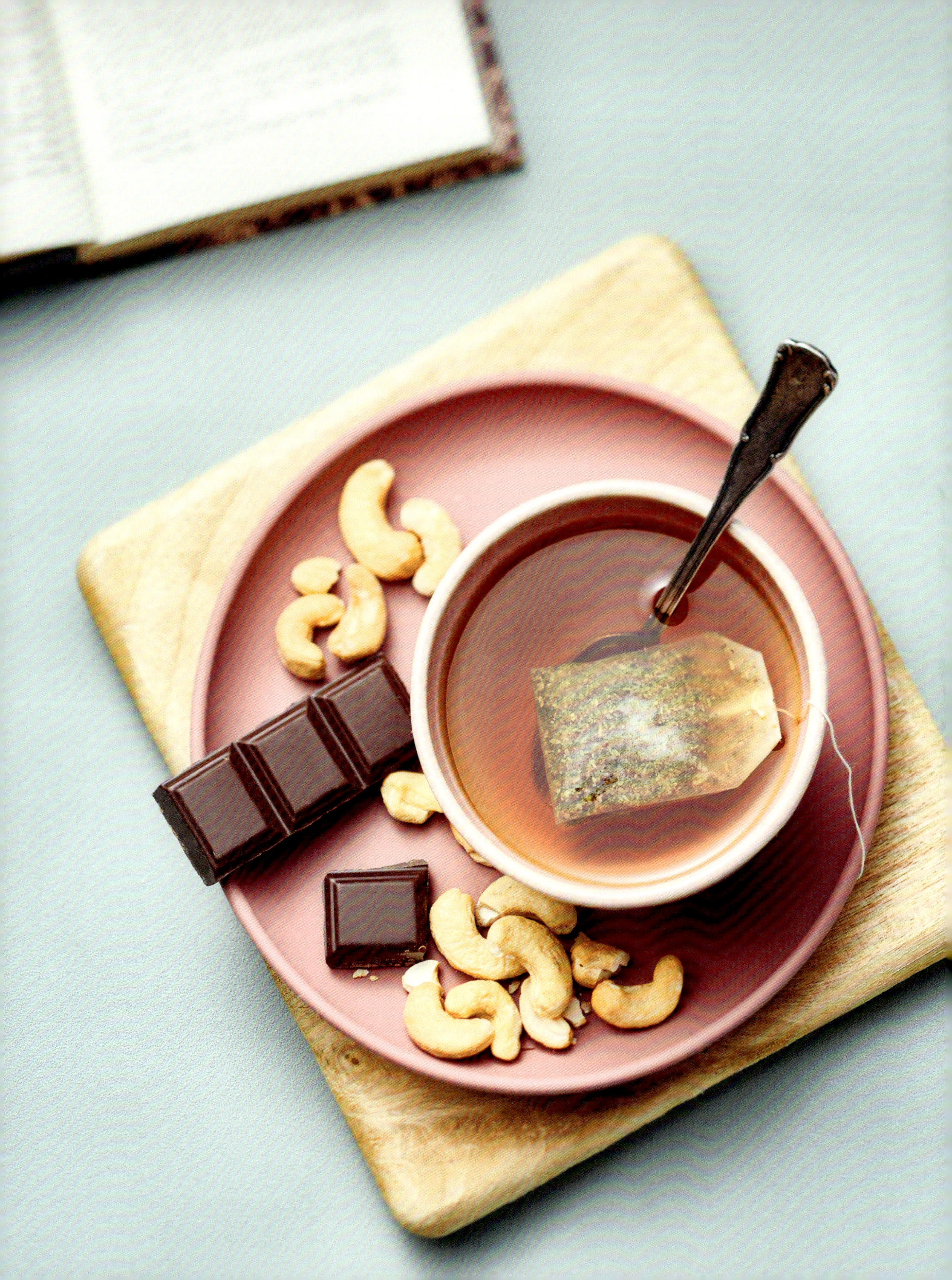

Relaxing Drinks for Sweet Dreams

Moon Milk with Ashwagandha

Serves 1
Prep: 5 minutes
Cook: 5 minutes

- 1 cup plant-based milk (almond, oat, or coconut)
- ½ teaspoon ashwagandha powder
- ½ teaspoon cinnamon
- Pinch nutmeg
- ½ teaspoon coconut oil
- 1 teaspoon honey or maple syrup (optional)

Moon milk is a traditional ayurvedic drink. The key ingredient in this recipe is ashwagandha, an adaptogenic plant that helps the body adapt to stress. Keep in mind that ashwagandha can act as a stimulant if the body needs a boost, so listen to your body's needs.

Heat the milk in a small saucepan over low heat. Add the ashwagandha, cinnamon, and nutmeg, then whisk together. Heat for around 5 minutes but do not let it boil. Remove from heat and add the coconut oil and honey (if using) before whisking again. Pour into a mug and enjoy 30 minutes before going to bed.

Golden Turmeric Latte

Serves 1
Prep: 5 minutes
Cook: 5 minutes

- 1 cup of plant-based milk (almond, coconut, or oat)
- 1 teaspoon turmeric paste (see recipe below)
- ½ teaspoon cinnamon
- Pinch black pepper
- ½ teaspoon coconut oil
- 1 teaspoon honey or maple syrup (optional)

Golden milk is a traditional Indian drink made with turmeric. It is known for its anti-inflammatory and calming properties. This drink is perfect for relaxing the body before sleep while reducing inflammation linked to menopause.

Heat the milk in a small saucepan over low heat. Add the turmeric paste, cinnamon, and pepper. Whisk together. Heat for 5 minutes without letting it boil. Remove from heat and add the coconut oil and honey (if using), then whisk again. Pour into a mug and enjoy 30 minutes before going to bed.

Turmeric Paste

Makes 1 jar
Prep: 5 minutes
Cook: 5 minutes
Keeps 2 weeks in the refrigerator

- ¼ cup ground turmeric
- ¼ cup ground ginger
- ¼ teaspoon black pepper

Combine all ingredients with ½ cup of water in a small saucepan. Heat over a low flame, stirring constantly, until the mixture forms a smooth paste (around 5 minutes). Let cool then transfer to an airtight glass jar.

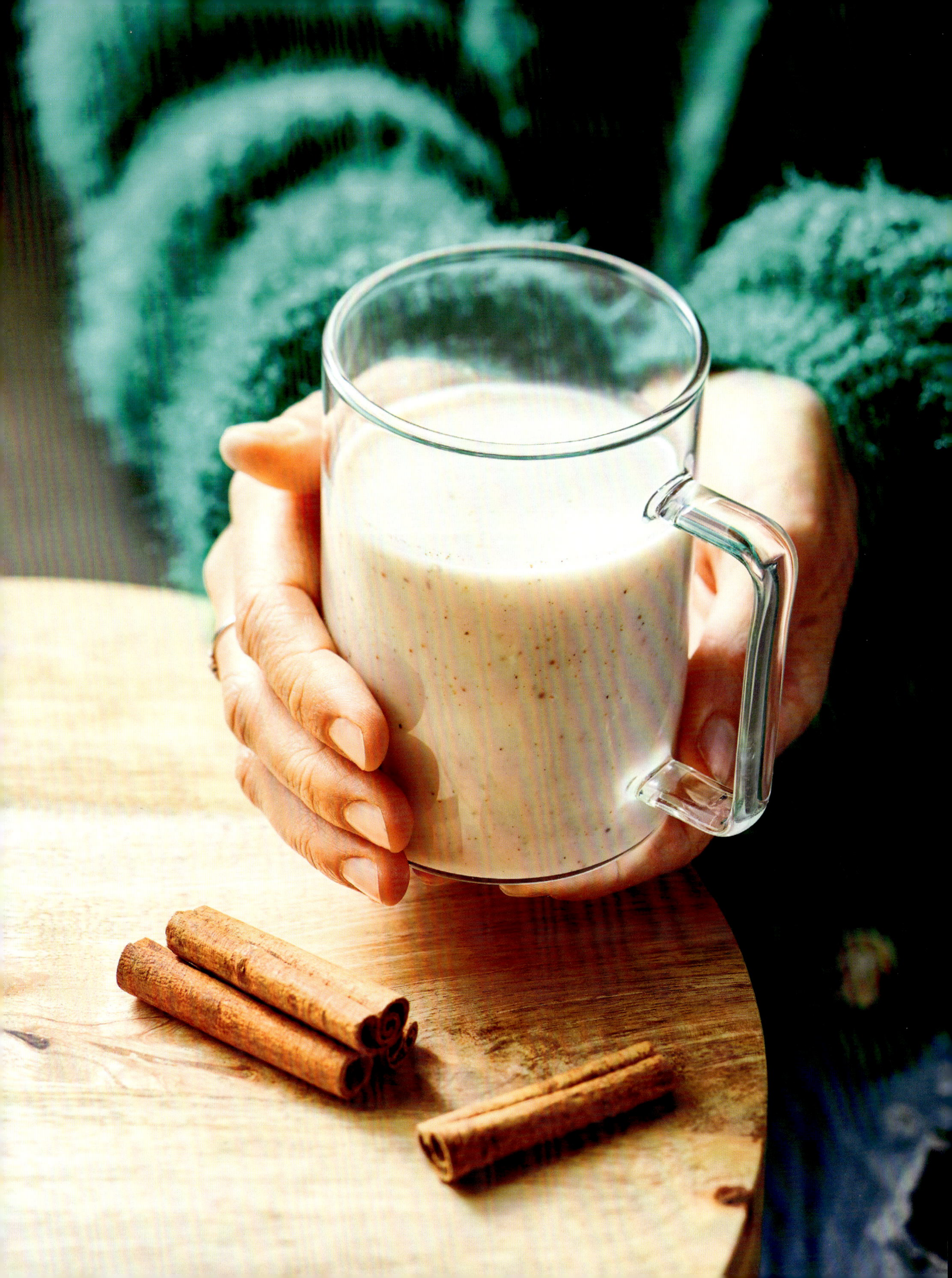

Herbal Teas to Take You to Dreamland

Serves 1
Prep: 5 to 7 minutes

Chamomile and Lemon Balm

1 teaspoon dried chamomile flowers

1 teaspoon dried lemon balm leaves

1 teaspoon honey (optional)

Chamomile and lemon balm are both plants that are known for their calming effect on the body. This tea is the perfect way to get ready for a night of restorative sleep.

Heat some water to around 175°F (80°C). Avoid bringing to a boil as this will break down the beneficial compounds in the plants. Sprinkle the chamomile flowers and lemon balm leaves into a mug. Pour over the water and cover before steeping for 5 to 7 minutes (covering the cup helps preserve the tea's natural benefits). Strain, add honey if desired, and enjoy 30 minutes to 1 hour before going to bed.

HOW IT HELPS YOUR BODY

Chamomile: Chamomile has a calming and mildly sedative effect on the body and helps relax the nervous system.

Lemon balm: This plant relieves anxiety and eases tension to help the body fall asleep naturally.

Passion Flower and Linden

1 teaspoon dried passion flower leaves

1 teaspoon dried linden flowers

This infusion combines passion flower, a plant known for its calming properties, with linden, which is wonderful for calming anxiety and tension.

Heat some water to around 175°F (80°C). Avoid bringing to a boil as this will break down the beneficial compounds in the plants. Sprinkle the passion flower leaves and linden flowers into a mug. Pour over the water and cover before steeping for 5 to 7 minutes (covering the cup helps preserve the tea's natural benefits). Strain and enjoy 30 minutes to 1 hour before going to bed.

HOW IT HELPS YOUR BODY

- **Passion flower:** This plant is rich in flavonoids, and its calming properties can help fight against stress-related insomnia.
- **Linden:** Linden acts as a mild sedative, eases nervous tension, and promotes deep sleep.

Valerian and Lavender

1 teaspoon dried valerian root

1 teaspoon dried lavender flowers

Valerian is a plant that is particularly effective for promoting deep, restorative sleep. In this recipe it is paired with another relaxing plant: lavender.

Heat some water to around 175°F (80°C). Avoid bringing to a boil as this will break down the beneficial compounds in the plants. Sprinkle the valerian root and lavender flowers into a mug. Pour over the water and cover before steeping for 5 to 7 minutes (covering the cup helps preserve the tea's natural benefits). Strain and enjoy 30 minutes to 1 hour before going to bed.

HOW IT HELPS YOUR BODY

- **Valerian:** This plant acts as a natural sedative. It reduces the time it takes to fall asleep and improves sleep quality.
- **Lavender:** Known for its calming properties, lavender reduces tension and anxiety to help the body fall asleep.

Lemon Balm, Orange Blossom, and Hops

1 teaspoon dried lemon balm leaves

1 teaspoon dried orange blossoms

1 teaspoon dried hop cones

This tea combines lemon balm, orange blossom, and hops for relaxation before a night of restorative sleep.

Heat some water to around 175°F (80°C). Avoid bringing to a boil as this will break down the beneficial compounds in the plants. Sprinkle the lemon balm, orange blossom, and hops into a mug. Pour over the water and cover before steeping for 5 to 7 minutes (covering the cup helps preserve the tea's natural benefits). Strain and enjoy 30 minutes to 1 hour before going to bed.

HOW IT HELPS YOUR BODY

- **Lemon balm:** Reduces anxiety and improves sleep quality.
- **Orange blossom:** Calms the nervous system and promotes relaxation.
- **Hops:** Excellent for reducing nighttime restlessness.

Lavender and Lemon Verbena

1 teaspoon dried lavender flowers

1 teaspoon dried lemon verbena leaves

1 slice of lemon (optional)

1 teaspoon maple syrup or honey (optional)

This tea combines the gentle calm of lavender with lemon verbena, which is perfect for calming the mind and easing muscle tension to promote deeper sleep.

Heat some water to around 175°F (80°C). Avoid bringing to a boil as this will break down the beneficial compounds in the plants. Sprinkle the lavender flowers and lemon verbena leaves in a mug. Pour over the water and cover before steeping for 5 to 7 minutes (covering the cup helps preserve the tea's natural benefits). Strain, add the lemon and honey if desired, and enjoy 30 minutes to 1 hour before going to bed.

HOW IT HELPS YOUR BODY

- **Lavender:** Helps reduce anxiety and tension to make falling asleep easier.
- **Lemon verbena:** Soothes nerve and muscle tension and promotes healthy digestion before sleep.

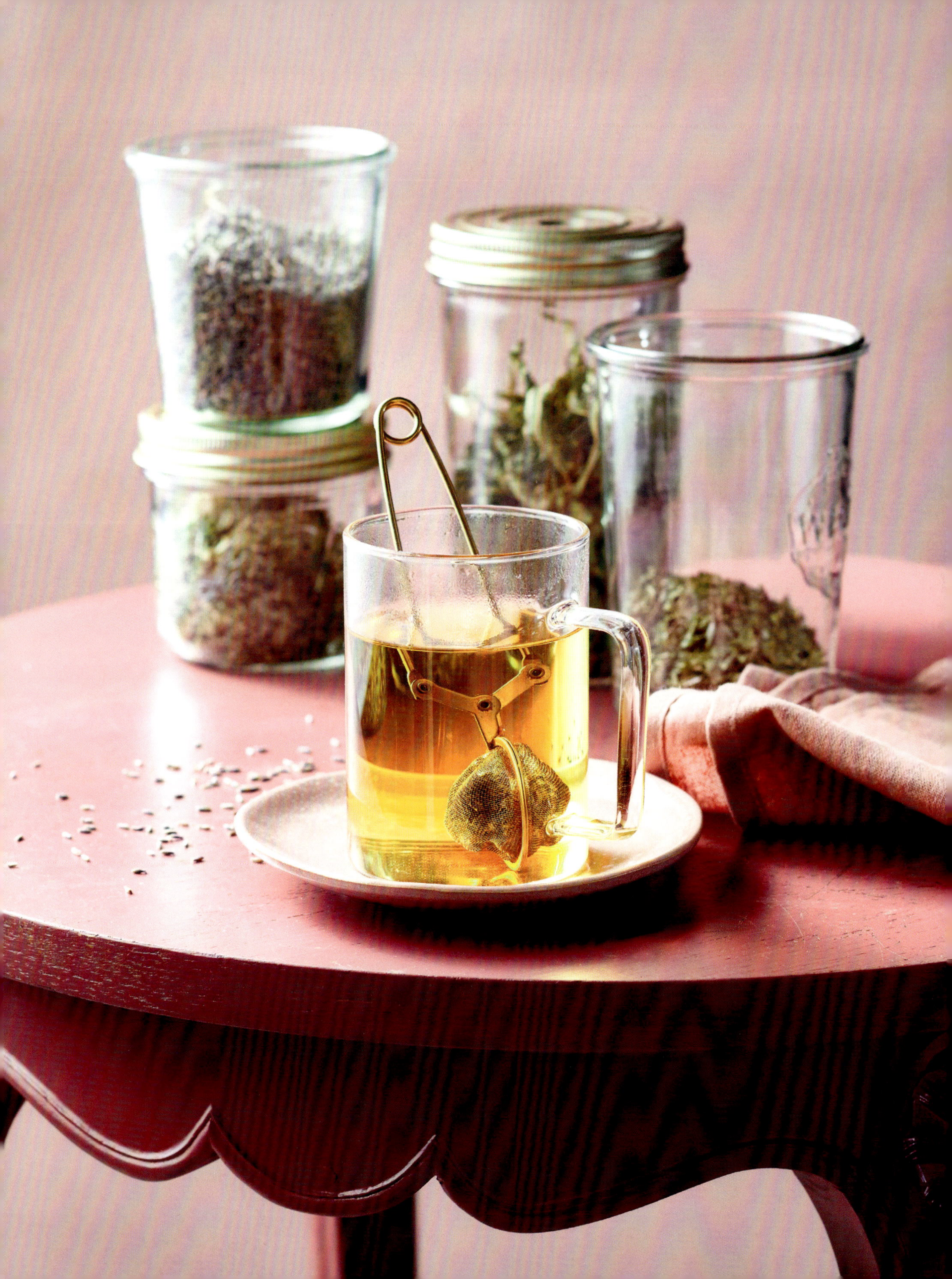

Recipes for Everyday Energy and Vitality

During menopause, hormonal fluctuations can cause a drop in energy, increased oxidative stress, and greater fatigue. This is when it becomes so important to support the body with targeted nutrients to keep your energy up. Antioxidants neutralize free radicals to protect cells, reduce inflammation, and promote energy production. They're found in fruits and vegetables and come in all kinds of colors—each one offering its own range of health benefits.

Antioxidants by Color

Red
Lycopene and Anthocyanins

Red antioxidants are particularly powerful when it comes to improving cardiovascular health and fighting inflammation. Lycopene (found in tomatoes and watermelon) helps protect the heart and maintain good circulation. Anthocyanins (found in berries) boost immunity and reduce inflammation.
Food sources: tomato, watermelon, grapefruit, red bell pepper, strawberry, cherry, raspberry, guava, papaya

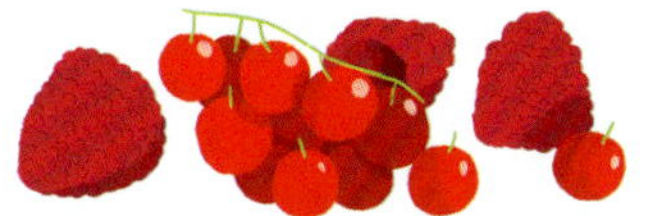

Orange and Yellow
Beta-Carotene and Vitamin C

Orange and yellow antioxidants are essential for eye health, energy production, and immunity. Beta-carotene (found in carrots and sweet potatoes) is converted to vitamin A in the body and supports eye health and cell function. Vitamin C (abundant in citrus fruit) plays a vital role in collagen production, cell repair, and reducing fatigue.
Food sources: carrots, mango, lemon, sweet potato, pumpkin, orange, apricot, dandelion, turmeric, pineapple, yellow bell pepper, banana

Green
Chlorophyll, Lutein, and Glucosinolates

Green antioxidants are excellent detoxifiers. They also protect the skin and help maintain stable energy levels. Chlorophyll brings oxygen to the cells and eliminates toxins while lutein protects vision and boosts cognitive health. Glucosinolates (found in cruciferous vegetables) detoxify the liver and support hormonal balance.
Food sources: spinach, broccoli, avocado, kale, parsley, Swiss chard, peas, arugula, watercress, fresh herbs

Blue and Purple
Anthocyanins and Flavonoids

Blue and purple antioxidants protect cells from oxidative stress and support brain function. Anthocyanins (abundant in berries and grapes) boost memory and concentration and promote better blood circulation.
Food sources: blueberry, blackberry, red grapes, acai, eggplant, red cabbage, cranberry, rhubarb, blackcurrant, sea buckthorn (these are the exception, they are orange!), elderberry, pomegranate

White and Brown
Allicin and Polyphenols

White and brown antioxidants may not be as brightly colored as the others, but they boast several impressive benefits for overall health. Allicin (found in garlic and onions) boosts immunity and improves circulation, making it easier to transport nutrients and oxygen to cells everywhere in the body. Polyphenols (found in nuts) promote a more effective anti-inflammatory response and reduce oxidative stress.
Food sources: garlic, onion, leek, mushrooms, nuts, dark chocolate

Chia Pudding with Berries

Serves 4
Prep: 10 minutes
Rest: 4 hours

13.5 fluid ounces (400 ml) plant-based milk (almond, oat, or coconut)

8.8 ounces (250 g) coconut yogurt

2.8 ounces (80 g) chia seeds

1 tablespoon maca powder (optional)

1 tablespoon maple syrup or honey (optional)

7 ounces (200 g) berries, fresh or frozen

Zest of 1 lemon

Fresh mint

RECIPE

Combine the milk and yogurt in a bowl. Add the chia seeds and stir well. Add the maca powder and maple syrup if using.

Refrigerate for at least 4 hours (or overnight) to allow the chia seeds to swell and thicken the pudding.

Right before serving, top with the berries, lemon zest, and mint leaves.

HOW IT HELPS YOUR BODY

- **Protein:** Chia seeds and coconut yogurt contain plant proteins to help maintain muscle mass and support energy.
- **Antioxidants:** Berries are rich in antioxidants, which fight against free radicals and reduce oxidative stress to promote beautiful skin and restore energy levels.
- **Omega-3 fatty acids:** Chia seeds contain omega-3s that support cardiovascular health and help fight the increased inflammation that comes with menopause.
- **Magnesium:** Plant-based milk and chia seeds are natural sources of magnesium, which helps regulate mood, reduce stress, and promotes healthy sleep.
- **Fiber:** Chia seeds and berries contain fiber to improve digestion and maintain balanced blood sugar levels for increased energy.

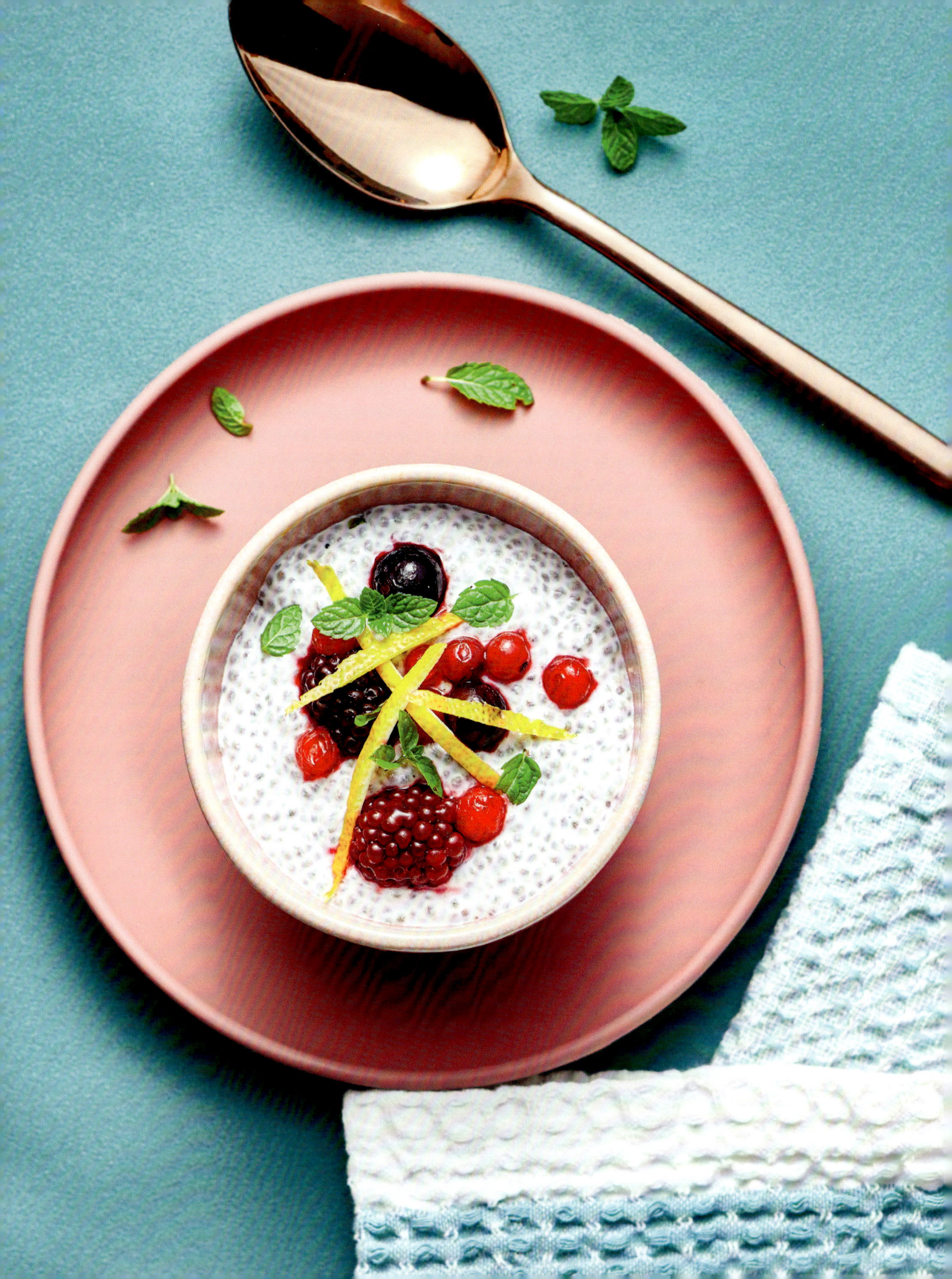

Acai Bowl

Serves 1
Prep: 5 minutes

3.5 ounces (100 g) frozen acai purée (available in health food stores)

½ banana, frozen or fresh

1.76 ounces (50 g) berries (strawberries, raspberries, or blueberries)

1 teaspoons chia seeds

3.5 fluid ounces (100 ml) plant-based milk (almond, coconut, oat)

1 teaspoon maple syrup

Toppings:

1 teaspoons unsweetened granola

Banana slices

1 tablespoon chopped cashews

1 teaspoon hemp seeds

Goji berries

Fresh mint

RECIPE

Add the acai purée, peeled banana, berries, chia seeds, and milk to a blender and blend until smooth and creamy. Pour into a bowl.

Add your choice of toppings and serve immediately.

HOW IT HELPS YOUR BODY

- **Antioxidants:** Acai and berries are rich in anthocyanins and polyphenols that protect cells from oxidative stress. This improves vitality and overall energy.
- **Fiber:** Chia seeds, berries, and granola provide a healthy dose of fiber to improve digestion and maintain stable blood sugar levels so you can avoid sudden drops in energy.
- **Magnesium:** Cashews and hemp seeds contain magnesium, which is essential for restorative seep, managing stress, and reducing menopause symptoms.
- **Omega-3 fatty acids:** Chia seeds and hemp seeds contain omega-3s that support hormonal health and reduce inflammation.
- **Plant protein:** Hemp seeds and cashews provide plant protein, which helps maintain muscle mass and energy.

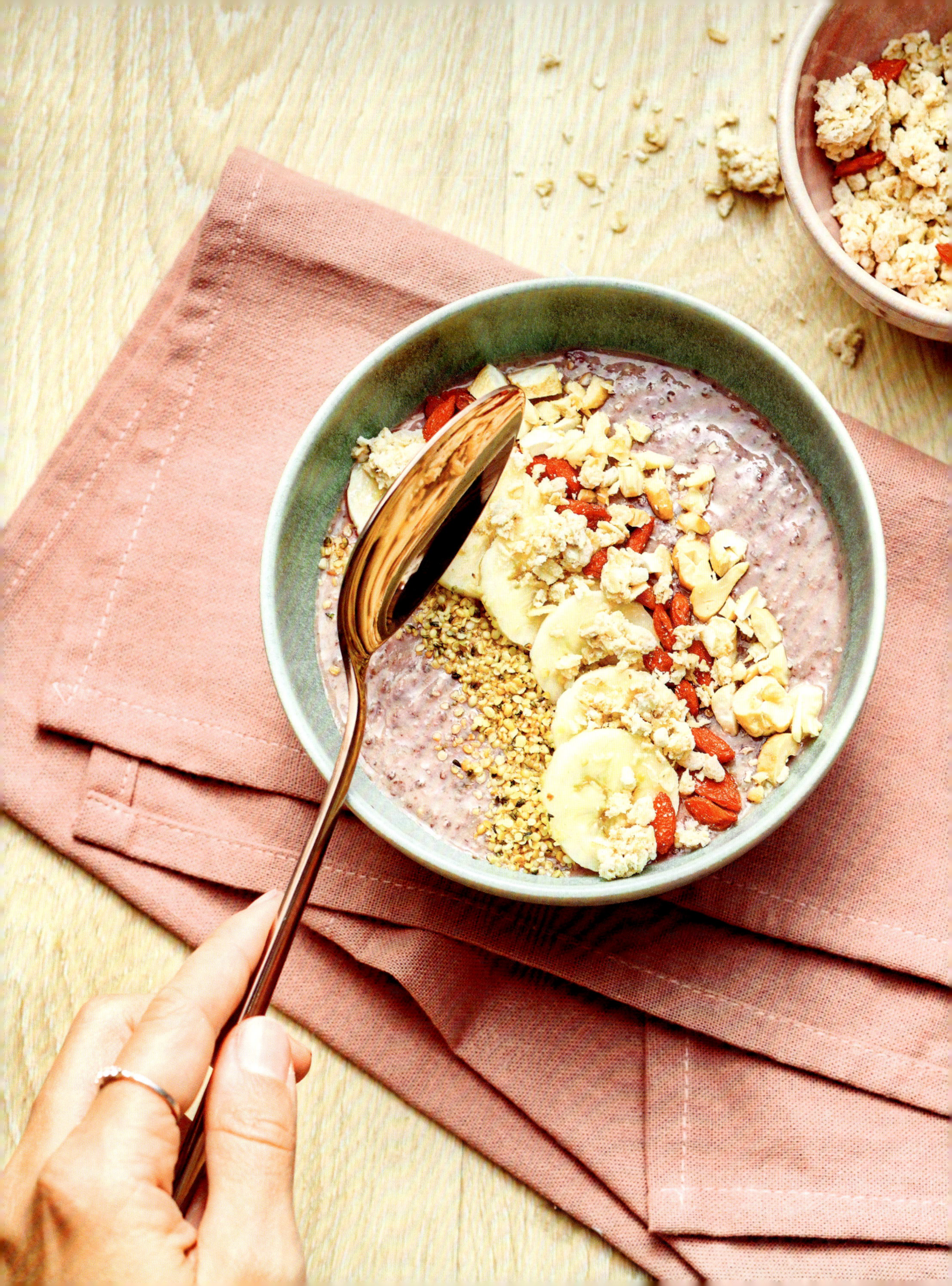

Berry Avocado Smoothie

Serves 1
Prep: 5 minutes

1 ripe avocado

5.3 ounces (150 g) berries, fresh or frozen

1 banana

6.75 fluid ounces (200 ml) plant-based milk (almond, coconut, or oat)

1 tablespoon chia seeds

RECIPE

Cut the avocado in half, remove the pit, and scoop out the flesh. Add to a blender along with the berries, peeled banana, milk, and chia seeds. Blend until smooth and creamy.

Pour into a glass and serve immediately.

HOW IT HELPS YOUR BODY

- **Antioxidants:** Berries are rich in antioxidants that help fight oxidative stress and boost vitality. They also support cardiovascular health and memory.
- **Fiber:** Chia seeds and bananas provide fiber to facilitate digestion and regulate blood sugar levels. This contributes to stable energy levels throughout the day.
- **Healthy fats:** Avocado and chia seeds are rich in omega-3 fatty acids and healthy fats. These are essential for soft, supple skin and hormonal health.
- **Magnesium:** Chia seeds and avocado contain magnesium, which plays a key role in restorative sleep, managing stress, and handling mood swings.
- **Potassium:** Avocado and bananas are good sources of potassium, which means that they help regulate fluid balance in the body and maintain healthy blood pressure. All of these things contribute to increased vitality.

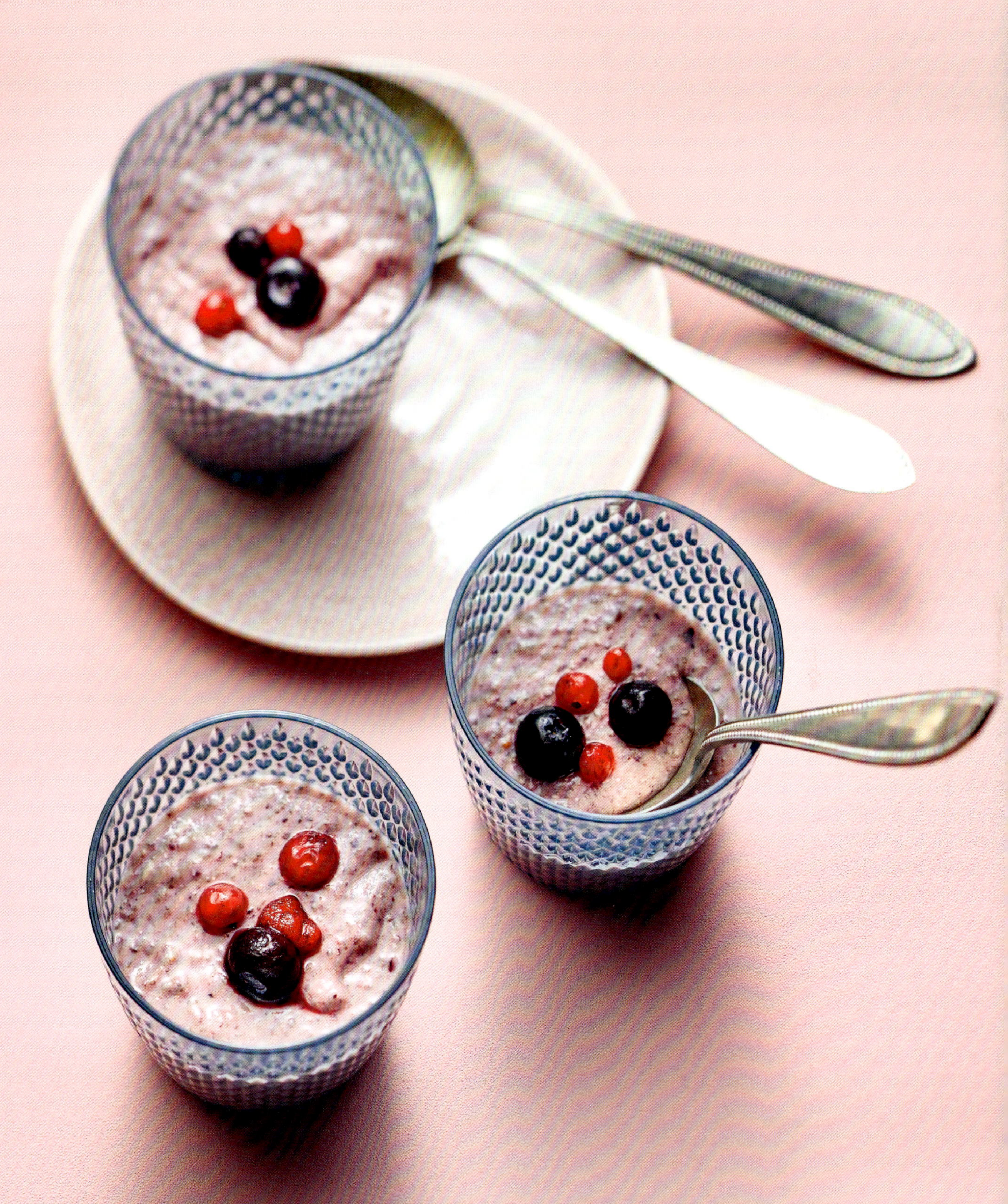

Recipe List

Ingredient Index

Recipe Index

Published originally under the title *Mes recettes pour une ménopause en douceur*

Skyhorse Publishing books may be purchased in bulk at special discounts for sales promotion, corporate gifts, fundraising, or educational purposes. Special editions can also be created to specifications. For details, contact the Special Sales Department, Skyhorse Publishing, 307 Fifth Avenue, 4th Floor, New York, NY 10016 or info@skyhorsepublishing.com.

Visit our website at www.skyhorsepublishing.com.

10 9 8 7 6 5 4 3 2 1

Library of Congress Cataloging-in-Publication Data on file.

Publisher: **Didier Férat**
Editorial Director: **Fanny Ecochard-Martin**
Editor: **Diane Monserat**
Translation: **Grace McQuillan**
Design and formatting: **Julia Philipps and Marina Delranc**
Photo-engraving: **Chromostyle**

Portrait on page 6: **Anaïs Darnay**

Print ISBN: 978-1-5107-8628-8
Ebook ISBN: 978-1-5107-8705-6

Printed in China